BASIC AND CLINICAL PHARMACOLOGY FOR MEDICAL GRADUATES

Syed Ahmed Hussain,
Junaid Tantray,
Ashish Kumar Sharma

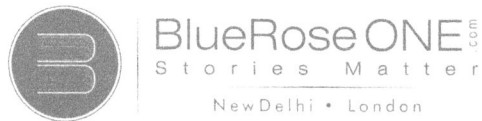

New Delhi • London

BLUEROSE PUBLISHERS
India | U.K.

Copyright © Syed Ahmed Hussain Junaid Tantray Ashish Kumar Sharma 2023

All rights reserved by author. No part of this publication may be reproduced, stored in a retrieval system or transmitted in any form or by any means, electronic, mechanical, photocopying, recording or otherwise, without the prior permission of the author. Although every precaution has been taken to verify the accuracy of the information contained herein, the publisher assume no responsibility for any errors or omissions. No liability is assumed for damages that may result from the use of information contained within.

BlueRose Publishers takes no responsibility for any damages, losses, or liabilities that may arise from the use or misuse of the information, products, or services provided in this publication.

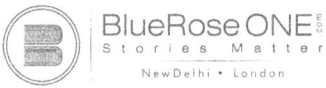

For permissions requests or inquiries regarding this publication,
please contact:

BLUEROSE PUBLISHERS
www.BlueRoseONE.com
info@bluerosepublishers.com
+91 8882 898 898
+4407342408967

ISBN: 978-93-5819-334-3

Cover design: Tahira
Typesetting: Namrata Saini

First Edition: November 2023

DEDICATED TO

- **The creator**
- **My Parents**
- **My wife**
- **My family**
- **My students for always challenging us**

Key Features of the Book:

- ✓ Comprehensive Coverage: We have carefully structured the content to cover both basic principles and advanced clinical applications, ensuring a solid foundation for medical students and professionals alike.
- ✓ Integration of Clinical Scenarios: Throughout the book, we have integrated real-world clinical scenarios to demonstrate how pharmacological knowledge is applied in actual medical practice. This approach bridges the gap between theory and practical application.
- ✓ Clear and Concise Explanations: Complex topics are explained in a reader-friendly language, with the use of illustrations, diagrams, and tables to enhance understanding.
- ✓ Updated Information: As the field of pharmacology is constantly evolving, we have taken great care to include the latest research findings and developments, ensuring that readers stay abreast of current trends and advancements.
- ✓ Self-Assessment Tools: To aid in the learning process, each chapter includes self-assessment questions and case studies, allowing readers to test their knowledge and problem-solving skills.

Contributions

Drugs used in gastrointestinal disorders	*Aminu Wada Musa* *B.Pharm Scholar*
Drugs acting on Clotting Disorders	*Nilesh Sharma, Pragya Pandey* *Pharm D Research Scholar*

PREFACE

Welcome to "Basic and Clinical Pharmacology for Medical Sciences." This book is designed to be a comprehensive and accessible resource for students and professionals in the medical field, providing a thorough understanding of the fundamental principles and practical applications of pharmacology.

Pharmacology plays a pivotal role in modern medicine, as it encompasses the study of how drugs interact with the human body to diagnose, prevent, and treat various diseases and conditions. In this book, we aim to demystify the complexities of pharmacology by presenting the subject matter in a clear and concise manner, making it easy for readers to grasp the core concepts and their clinical implications. We hope that "Basic and Clinical Pharmacology for Medical Sciences" will serve as an invaluable companion on your journey to becoming proficient in pharmacology. Whether you are a medical student embarking on your educational path or a seasoned healthcare professional seeking to reinforce your knowledge, this book is intended to be your reliable guide in understanding the principles and applications of pharmacology in the realm of medical sciences.

Our heartfelt gratitude goes to all the contributors and reviewers who have dedicated their time and expertise to enrich the content of this book. Your commitment to advancing medical education is greatly appreciated.

We sincerely hope that you find this book informative, engaging and a source of inspiration in your pursuit of medical knowledge and excellence in patient care.

Syed Ahmed Hussain
Junaid Tantray
Ashish Kumar Sharma

FORWARD

Dear Esteemed Students, Faculty, and Medical Professionals,

I am honored to introduce "Basic and Clinical Pharmacology for Medical Sciences," a comprehensive and essential resource that embodies our commitment to excellence in medical education and research.

As the President and CEO of **AGA ACADEMY** I take great pride in witnessing the publication of this exemplary book, which has been carefully curated to cater to the needs of our esteemed medical community. "Basic and Clinical Pharmacology for Medical Sciences" is a testament to our dedication to providing our students and faculty with the highest standard of educational materials. It's a joint venture between AGA Academy Calgary and Faculties of NIMS Institute of Pharmacy, NIMS University Rajasthan Jaipur

The field of pharmacology plays a crucial role in modern medicine, shaping the way we diagnose, prevent, and treat various diseases and conditions. Through this book, our esteemed faculty and researchers have collaborated to present a cohesive and detailed understanding of pharmacology's core principles and its practical applications.

I extend my gratitude to the talented team of authors, editors, and reviewers who have poured their expertise and dedication into producing this invaluable resource. Their commitment to advancing medical knowledge is evident in each chapter, making the book an indispensable guide for medical students, researchers, and healthcare professionals alike. Key Features of the Book includes Comprehensive Coverage, Real-World Application, Clarity and Conciseness, and Cutting-Edge Information. Together, we will continue to advance the frontiers of medical knowledge and make a lasting impact on patient care and public health.

Congratulations to all those involved in bringing this book to fruition. Your hard work and dedication are truly commendable.

With warm regards,
Abby Villanueva
President and CEO
Calgary, Alberta, Canada

TABLE OF CONTENTS

General Pharmacology 1
Drug used in Cardiology Hypertension and Related Pathologies 34
Drugs used in Lipid Disorders- Anti-Hyperlipidemia - 62
Drugs for Neuro-Psychiatry Drugs Working on CNS 72
Autacoids Antagonists 98
Pharmacology of Drugs Acting on Renal System: Antidiuretics 105
Drugs Affecting Respiratory System 116
Drugs Acting on Gastrointestinal Tract 123
Drugs used in Gastrointestinal Disorders 134
Drugs Affecting The Biliary System:- 148
Drugs Acting on Cns 156
Anti Viral Drug Classification 159
Anti-HIV Drugs 165
Drugs Acting on Clotting Disorders 189
Antibiotics 195
Agents used for Treatment of Fungus Infections 218
Agents used for Treatment of Tuberculosis 230
Pharmacovigilance 236

GENERAL PHARMACOLOGY

(A) Introduction, definition and scope of Pharmacology

DEFINITION OF PHARMACOLOGY

Pharmacology is the study of the therapeutic value and/or potential toxicity of chemical agents on biological systems.

It targets every aspect of the mechanisms for the chemical actions of both traditional and novel therapeutic agents.

Two important and interrelated areas are: pharmacokinetics and pharmacodynamic

Drug: According to WHO, drugs are substances that are used to prevent, diagnose, and treat diseases or medical conditions. They can be of natural or synthetic origin and may have various physiological effects when administered to humans or animals.

Drugs can be classified into different categories based on their intended use and potential effects, such as:

- **Medicinal drugs**: Pharmaceuticals that are used to treat, cure, prevent, or alleviate medical conditions and diseases. These can include over-the-counter medications, prescription drugs, and vaccines.
- **Recreational drugs:** Substances used for non-medical purposes, primarily to alter one's mood, perception, or consciousness. Examples include alcohol, cannabis, cocaine, and ecstasy.
- **Performance-enhancing drugs**: Substances used to enhance athletic performance or physical abilities. This category includes anabolic steroids, human growth hormone (HGH), and stimulants.

- ➤ **Illicit drugs**: Drugs that are illegal to possess, manufacture, or distribute, usually due to their potential for abuse and harm. Examples include heroin, methamphetamine, and certain hallucinogens.
- ➤ **Prescription drugs**: Medications that can only be legally obtained with a prescription from a licensed healthcare professional.

Pharmacokinetics (what body does with the drug) deals with the absorption, distribution, and excretion of drugs. Pharmacokinetics is a branch of pharmacology that deals with the study of how the body processes drugs. It focuses on understanding the movement of drugs within the body, including their absorption, distribution, metabolism, and excretion, often referred to by the acronym "ADME."

Pharmacodynamic (**what drug does with the body**) are the study of the molecular, biochemical, and physiological effects of drugs on cellular systems and their mechanisms of action. Pharmacodynamics is a branch of pharmacology that deals with the study of how drugs interact with the body at the molecular, cellular, and systemic levels to produce their pharmacological effects. It focuses on understanding the relationship between drug concentration and its physiological and biochemical effects on the body.

Pharmacy: Pharmacy is a healthcare profession that deals with the preparation, dispensing, and proper use of medications. Pharmacists are trained professionals who work in various settings, including community pharmacies, hospitals, clinics, and other healthcare facilities. They play a critical role in promoting health and ensuring the safe and effective use of medications by patients.

Therapeutics: It is the aspect of medicine concerned with the treatment of diseases. Therapeutics, also known as medical therapy or treatment, refers to the application of medical interventions to manage, alleviate, or cure diseases, medical conditions, or health problems in patients. The goal of therapeutics is to improve a patient's health and well-being through various medical approaches, including the use of medications, surgical procedures, physical therapies, and lifestyle modifications.

Chemotherapy: It deals with the treatment of infectious disease/cancer with chemical compounds that cause relatively selective damage to the infecting organism/cancer cells. Chemotherapy, often abbreviated as chemo, is a form of medical treatment that uses powerful medications to treat cancer and certain other conditions. It is a systemic therapy, meaning that the drugs circulate throughout the body, affecting both the cancerous cells and some normal cells. The primary goal of chemotherapy is to destroy or inhibit the growth and division of cancer cells, leading to tumor shrinkage or elimination.

Toxicology*:* It is study of poisons, their action, detection, prevention, and the treatment of poisoning. Toxicology is a scientific discipline that studies the adverse effects of chemical, physical, or biological agents on living organisms, including humans, animals, and plants. It is a multidisciplinary field that combines knowledge from biology, chemistry, pharmacology, environmental science, and medicine to understand the mechanisms by which toxic substances interact with living systems and how to manage or prevent their harmful effects.

Essential Medicines*:* Essential medicines, as defined by the World Health Organization, are the medicines that "satisfy the priority health care needs of the population". These are the medications to which people should have constant and adequate access. The prices should be within reach of the majority of people. In 1977, the first Essential Medicines List was released, followed by the first Essential Medicines List for Children in 2007. Iron and folic acid preparations for pregnant anaemia, antitubular medications such as isoniazid, rifampicin, pyranzinamide, Ethambutol, and others are examples.

Clinical Pharmacology: Clinical pharmacology is **the study of drugs in humans**. It has a broad scope, from the discovery of new target molecules, to the effects of drug usage in whole populations. Clinical pharmacologists are physicians, pharmacists, and scientists whose focus is developing and understanding new drug therapies.

Orphan Drugs: An orphan drug is a pharmaceutical agent developed to treat medical conditions which, because they are so rare, would not be profitable to produce without government assistance. The conditions are referred to as orphan diseases. The Orphan Drug Act was passed in 1983 to give drug companies incentives to develop treatments for rare diseases. E.g. Digoxin antibody (for digoxin toxicity).

Pharmacovigilance: Pharmacovigilance is the science and activities relating to the detection, assessment, understanding and prevention of adverse effects or any other medicine/vaccine related problem. All medicines and vaccines undergo rigorous testing for safety and efficacy through clinical trials before they are authorized for use.

Receptor: Receptors are specific proteins or molecules on the surface of cells or within cells that interact with drugs and initiate a biological response. Drug-receptor interactions play a crucial role in pharmacodynamics.

Receptors are specialized proteins or molecules located on the surface of cells or inside cells that bind to specific signaling molecules, such as hormones, neurotransmitters, or drugs. When these signaling molecules bind to their respective receptors, it triggers a series of cellular responses or biochemical pathways, leading to various physiological effects in the body. There are several families or types of receptors, classified based on their structure, mechanism of action, and the type of signaling molecule they bind to. Some of the major receptor families include:

The basics

1.1.2 History and of pharmacology

The history of pharmacology is a fascinating journey that dates back thousands of years. Here are some key milestones in the development of pharmacology:

Ancient Times: The use of natural substances for medicinal purposes can be traced back to ancient civilizations such as the Sumerians, Egyptians, and Chinese. Herbal remedies and plant-based substances were commonly employed to treat various ailments.

Ancient Greek and Roman Period: In ancient Greece, scholars like Hippocrates emphasized the importance of observation and documentation of drug effects. The Greek physician Dioscorides compiled one of the earliest pharmacological texts, "De Materia Medica," which described hundreds of medicinal plants.

Middle Ages: During the Middle Ages, much of the knowledge from ancient civilizations was preserved and further developed by Islamic scholars in the Middle East. The Persian physician Avicenna wrote extensively on pharmacology and medicine in his renowned medical encyclopedia, "The Canon of Medicine."

Renaissance and Early Modern Period: The Renaissance era saw the resurgence of interest in anatomy, physiology, and the study of the human body. Paracelsus, a Swiss physician and alchemist, challenged traditional medicine and emphasized the importance of using chemicals for therapeutic purposes.

19th Century: The 19th century brought significant advancements in pharmacology, particularly with the isolation and identification of active compounds from plants. For instance, morphine, quinine, and digitalis were isolated and used for medical purposes.

Late 19th and 20th Centuries: The development of synthetic chemistry revolutionized pharmacology, leading to the production of various new drugs. This era saw the emergence of pharmacological research laboratories and the establishment of pharmacology as a distinct scientific discipline.

Pharmacokinetics and Pharmacodynamics: In the 20th century, researchers made significant strides in understanding the absorption, distribution, metabolism, and excretion of drugs (pharmacokinetics) and the mechanisms by which drugs exert their effects (pharmacodynamics).

Drug Regulations: With the increasing use of drugs and concerns about safety, drug regulations and legislation were introduced to ensure the safety and efficacy of medications. Organizations like the U.S. Food and Drug Administration (FDA) were established to oversee drug approvals and monitor post-marketing safety.

Molecular Pharmacology: Advances in molecular biology and genetics have further enriched pharmacology. Molecular pharmacologists study drug-receptor interactions at the molecular level and develop targeted therapies based on specific molecular pathways.

Personalized Medicine: In recent years, pharmacology has moved toward personalized medicine, where treatments are tailored to an individual's genetic makeup and specific disease characteristics.

Today, pharmacology continues to evolve rapidly, integrating various scientific disciplines and cutting-edge technologies to develop safer and more effective medications for the benefit of global healthcare. Researchers in pharmacology play a vital role in drug discovery, drug development, and the understanding of drug interactions and mechanisms of action. It's fascinating to learn how the medicinal area unit was found and evolved. Historically, this was usually backed either by lore or careful observation (e.g. digitalis leaf, penicillin). Nowadays, a novel pharmaceutical is mostly developed by an organic chemist using a pill roller, based on fundamental data about major molecular targets. Biological screens are sometimes used to select chemical compounds for optimal medical specialty action. Medication data sources recommend providing clinically useful data on any aspect of drug use for individual patients as well as broad data on how to best use medicine for populations. The first drug data centre, located at the University of Kentucky medical centre, was established in 1962.

1.1.3 SOURCE OF DRUGS

Drugs fall into three main categories: natural, semisynthetic, and synthetic. Natural drugs are sourced from various elements like plants, animals, minerals, and microorganisms. Semisynthetic drugs originate from natural sources and undergo chemical alterations. Synthetic drugs, on the other hand, are entirely created through artificial chemical synthesis.

The different sources of drugs:

1. Plants:
   a) Alkaloids are nitrogen containing compounds, e.g. morphine, atropine, quinine, reserpine, ephedrine.
   b) Glycosides contain sugar group in combination with nonsugar through ether linkage, e.g. digoxin, digitoxin.
   c) Volatile oils have aroma. They are useful for relieving pain (clove oil), as carminative (eucalyptus oil), flavouring agent (peppermint oil), etc.
   d) Resins are sticky organic compounds obtained from pants as exudate, e.g. tincture benzoin (antiseptic).

2. Animals: Insulin, heparin, antisera.

3. Minerals: Ferrous sulphate, magnesium sulphate.

4. Microorganisms: Penicillin G, streptomycin, griseofulvin (antimicrobial agents), streptokinase (fibrinolytic).

5. Semisynthetic: Hydromorphone, hydrocodone.

6. Synthetic: Most of the drugs used today are synthetic, e.g. aspirin, paracetamol.

Drugs are also produced by genetic engineering (DNA recombinant technology), ¢.g. human insulin, human growth hormone and hepatitis B vaccine.

1.1.4 Source of drug information

Pharmacopoeia: An aggregation, formulary, or pharmacopoeia, in its fashionable technical sense, could be a book containing directions for the identification of compound medicines, and revealed by the authority of a government or a medical or pharmaceutical society.

Monographs are descriptions of preparations. Indian Pharmacopoeia(IP), British Pharmacopoeia(BP), European Pharmacopoeia(EP), and United States Pharmacopoeia(USP) are a few of the aggregate area unit (USP).Other sources are Textbooks, newsletters, journals,

- ✓ Newsletters, microfilm reader,
- ✓ Optical discs,
- ✓ Laptop systems
- ✓ Tertiary resources >>>Secondary resources >>>Primary resources secondary sources consists of reviews of primary reports.

These give a private perspective of the literature and would possibly} embrace comments on how the author might apply the knowledge in applying.

- ✓ Medline
- ✓ International Pharmaceutical abstracts
- ✓ Chemical Abstracts
- ✓ IOWA drug data Service
- ✓ DRUGDEX
- ✓ Martindale
- ✓ POISINDEX

1.1.5 CONCEPT OF ESSENTIAL MEDICINES

Definition

Essential medicines are those that satisfy the priority health care needs of the majority of population The concept of essential medicines is a key component of public health and healthcare systems worldwide. It was first introduced by the World Health Organization (WHO) in 1977 with the aim of promoting equitable access to safe, effective, and affordable medications for all individuals, particularly in resource-limited settings. Essential medicines are considered the minimum pharmaceutical needs that should be available in a healthcare system to address the most important health conditions and meet the primary healthcare needs of the population.

Key aspects of the concept of essential medicines include:

- **Essential Medicines List (EML):** The WHO maintains an Essential Medicines List, which includes a selection of drugs considered essential for addressing major public health issues. The list is regularly updated and divided into two categories: the Core List, which contains the most important and necessary medicines for a basic healthcare system, and the Complementary List, which includes additional medicines for more specialized needs.
- **Rational Use of Medicines:** The concept of essential medicines emphasizes the rational use of medications. This means that healthcare professionals should prescribe and use essential medicines based on evidence-based clinical guidelines, taking into account the safety, efficacy, and cost-effectiveness of the drugs.
- **Affordability and Accessibility**: Essential medicines are intended to be affordable and accessible to all individuals, regardless of their economic status. By focusing on cost-effective treatments, the concept seeks to reduce financial barriers to essential medications and improve health outcomes.
- **Promoting Quality Assurance**: Essential medicines should meet high-quality standards to ensure their safety and efficacy. Quality assurance measures include proper manufacturing, storage, and distribution of medications.
- **Global Health Perspective**: The concept of essential medicines is relevant not only for individual countries but also for global health efforts. Ensuring access to essential medicines is a crucial component of achieving universal health coverage and meeting the Sustainable Development Goals (SDGs) related to health and well-being.
- **Policy and Advocacy:** Governments, healthcare institutions, and international organizations play a vital role in implementing policies and programs that support the availability and accessibility of essential medicines. Advocacy efforts raise awareness about the importance of essential medicines and promote their integration into healthcare systems.

1.1.6 Criteria for selection of essential medicines

The process of choosing essential medicines is intricate, requiring a thoughtful evaluation of multiple factors to guarantee that the selected drugs align with the healthcare requirements of the populace and contribute to enhanced health results. The World Health Organization (WHO) has furnished directives for the selection of essential medicines, and each nation has the flexibility to tailor these guidelines to suit its unique healthcare landscape. Below are some prevalent criteria employed in the selection of essential medications:

Disease Burden: Essential medicines should target the most prevalent and significant health conditions affecting the population. The selection process considers the burden of diseases such as infectious diseases, chronic conditions, and other prevalent health issues.

Efficacy and Safety: The medicines selected must have proven efficacy and safety profiles, based on reliable scientific evidence from clinical trials and other sources. The benefits of the medicines should outweigh the potential risks and adverse effects.

Cost-effectiveness: Essential medicines are chosen with consideration for their cost-effectiveness. The goal is to maximize health benefits while optimizing resource allocation. Medicines that provide the most significant health impact at a reasonable cost are prioritized.

Public Health Impact: Medicines that have a substantial impact on public health, such as vaccines for infectious diseases or treatments for life-threatening conditions, are given priority in the selection process.

Accessibility: Essential medicines should be available and accessible to all segments of the population, especially in resource-limited settings. Consideration is given to factors such as affordability, availability, and geographical distribution of the medicines.

Therapeutic Need and Unmet Needs: The selection process considers the therapeutic needs of the population and aims to address unmet medical needs, especially for conditions where no effective treatment currently exists.

Health System Capacity: Essential medicines are selected based on the capacity of the healthcare system to procure, store, and distribute them effectively. The feasibility of integrating the medicines into the existing healthcare infrastructure is an essential consideration.

Local Health Policies and Guidelines: The selection of essential medicines aligns with national or regional health policies, treatment guidelines, and formularies. This ensures consistency with the healthcare priorities of the country.

Formulation and Dosage: Medicines that are available in appropriate formulations (e.g., oral, injectable, etc.) and suitable dosages for different age groups and patient populations are preferred.

Consensus and Stakeholder Involvement: The selection process involves consultation and collaboration with various stakeholders, including healthcare professionals, policymakers, patient advocacy groups, and international health organizations, to ensure broad consensus and support.

By considering these criteria, countries can develop a list of essential medicines that serves as the foundation for a well-functioning healthcare system, improving access to safe and effective treatments and contributing to better health outcomes for their populations.

1.1.7 Drug Nomenclature

Drug nomenclature refers to the systematic naming and classification of drugs to create a standardized and universally recognized system for identifying medications. Proper drug nomenclature is essential for clear communication among healthcare professionals, researchers, and regulatory authorities worldwide.

There are three primary aspects of drug nomenclature:

1. **Chemical Name:** The chemical name of a drug is the most precise and scientifically descriptive name. It reflects the drug's chemical structure and composition, providing valuable information to chemists and researchers. The chemical name can be lengthy and complex, making it less practical for everyday use.

Example: (6R-trans)-6-(1,3-benzodioxol-5-yl)-2,3,6,7,12,12a-hexahydro-2-methyl-pyrazino[1',2':1,6]pyrido[3,4-b]indole-1,4-dione (Chemical name of the antidepressant drug Sertraline)

2. **Generic Name (Non-proprietary Name):** The generic name, also known as the non-proprietary name, is a simplified and universally recognized name for a drug. It is typically shorter and more manageable than the chemical name. Generic names are assigned by health authorities, such as the World Health Organization (WHO) or the United States Adopted Names (USAN) Council.

Example: Sertraline (Generic name of the antidepressant drug)

3. **Brand Name (Trade Name):** The brand name, also known as the trade name or proprietary name, is the name given to a drug by a pharmaceutical company when marketing the medication. Brand names are unique to each manufacturer and are used for commercial purposes. Different manufacturers may market the same drug under different brand names.

Example: Zoloft® (Brand name of the antidepressant drug marketed by Pfizer)

It's important to note that a single drug can have multiple brand names from different manufacturers, but it will have only one generic name, which is the same for all formulations. Standardization of drug nomenclature is crucial to avoid confusion and ensure accurate prescribing, dispensing, and administration of medications. Healthcare professionals typically use the generic name when prescribing drugs to promote cost-effective prescribing and avoid confusion related to multiple brand names. The brand name is used mainly for marketing and patient identification purposes.

Routes of Administration

The drug administration route can be straightforwardly described as the approach through which a medication is introduced into the body with the intent of diagnosing, preventing, curing, or addressing a range of diseases and health issues. To achieve the intended therapeutic outcome, a medication must come into contact with the tissues of organs and cells, and it must be administered effectively to facilitate this interaction.

The drug bioavailability, which influences the start and duration of the pharmacological impact, is directly influenced by the method of administration. Many factors can influence the route of administration you choose, including:

I. Convenience

II. State of the patient
III. The desired onset of action
IV. Patient's co-operation
V. the nature of the drug as some drugs may be effective by one route only e.g., insulin
VI. Age of the patient
VII. Effect of gastric pH, digestive enzymes and first-pass metabolism

The various routes of administration are classified into a local route and systemic route. The local route is the simplest mode of administration of a drug at the site where the desired action is required. When the systemic absorption of a drug is desired, medications are usually administered by two main routes: the enteral route and the parenteral route.

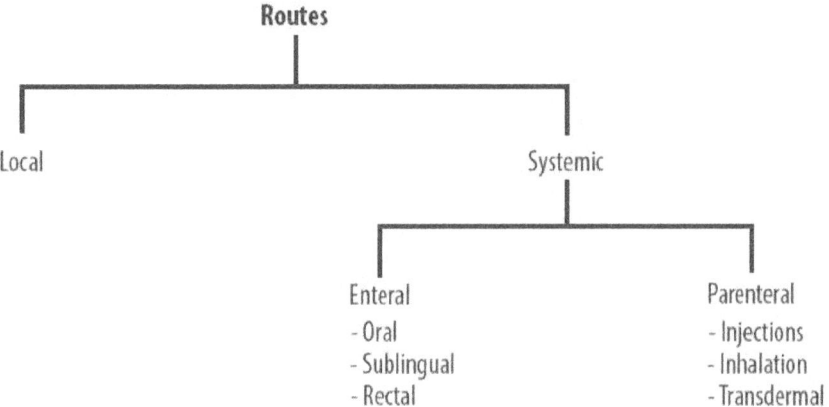

Classification of various routes of drug administration

The enteral route, which includes oral, sublingual, and rectal delivery, involves medication absorption through the gastrointestinal tract. The parenteral route, on the other hand, includes injection methods (e.g., intravenous, intramuscular, subcutaneous, etc.), inhalational, and transdermal routes that do not include drug absorption via the gastrointestinal tract (par = surrounding, enteral =gastrointestinal). Different routes of drug administration

1. Oral route
2. Sublingual/ Buccal route
3. Rectal route

4. Topical route

5. Transdermal route

6. Inhalational route/ pulmonary route

7. Injection route

1. Oral route

The most commonly employed method for administering drugs is through the oral route. When feasible, it is the preferred choice for drug administration due to its convenience and cost-effectiveness. In oral drug administration, medications are placed in the mouth and then swallowed.

In the case of oral administration, many drugs are efficiently absorbed from the gastrointestinal tract, provided their physicochemical properties are suitable. Some drugs are taken orally primarily for their localized effects within the gastrointestinal system, such as antacids for heartburn and ezetimibe for reducing cholesterol absorption. For oral drugs to be effective, they must withstand the acidic conditions of the stomach and traverse the intestinal lining before entering the bloodstream. Common oral dosage forms include tablets, capsules, suspensions, solutions, and emulsions.

Note: - Insulin cannot be given orally because it destroys digestive juices in the stomach.

Advantages of oral route of drug administration

1. It is the simplest, most convenient, and safest means of drug administration.
2. It is convenient for repeated and prolonged use.
3. It can be self-administered and pain-free.
4. It is economical since it does not involve the patient in extra cost. Where the drug is a solid e.g., tablet and capsule, the patient needs just one or two cups of water, which in most cases is freely available. If the drug is in liquid form, nothing is needed except a measuring tool that comes with the drug in most cases.
5. No sterile precautions are needed.
6. Danger of acute drug reaction is minimal.

Disadvantages of oral route of drug administration

1. It is not suitable for emergencies as the onset of action of orally administered drugs is relatively slow.
2. It can only be used in conscious patients and those patients who can swallow.
3. It requires patient cooperation or compliance, especially for outpatients.

It is not suitable for:

A. unpalatable and highly irritant drugs
B. drugs that are destroyed by gastric acid and digestive juices (e.g., insulin)
C. drugs with extensive first-pass metabolism (e.g. lignocaine, imipramine)
D. Patients with severe vomiting and diarrhoea.
E. Oral route of drug administration is sometimes inefficient as absorption is in most cases irregular and incomplete.
F. Changes in drug solubility can result from reactions with other materials present in the gastrointestinal tract e.g., the interference of absorption of tetracyclines through the formation of insoluble complexes with calcium, which can be available from dairy products or formulation additives.

2. Sublingual/ Buccal route

The medicine is put under the tongue (sublingual route) or between the gums and the inner lining of the cheek in this mode of administration (buccal route). The medicine is allowed to dissolve in both circumstances, avoiding ingesting as much as possible. The drug is rapidly absorbed into circulation through the mucosa, bypassing the portal circulation and, as a result, the liver's first-pass metabolism.

When the medication is destroyed or partially inactivated in the stomach if taken, and more immediate action is necessary, the sublingual and buccal routes are useful. Bitter medications, on the other hand, are not suitable for these routes.

Nitro-glycerine (glyceryl trinitrate), buprenorphine, and des amino-oxytocin are examples of medications that are delivered by sublingual and buccal methods.Advantages of buccal and sublingual routes of drug administration

Some advantages of administering drugs through the oral mucosa are:

1. A rapid onset of the therapeutic effect is achieved, not only by the high blood supply of the area but also by the lack of gastrointestinal (GI) factors that delay absorption (gastric emptying, presence of food, gastric disease, etc.).
2. Portal circulation is avoided, which allows for improving the bioavailability of a drug (regarding the oral route) avoiding intestinal and first-pass hepatic metabolism.
3. The active ingredient is not exposed to the aggressive GI medium, the reason why it is possible for the buccal administration of some drugs (e.g. peptides) that would otherwise be degraded by the GI pH or enzymes.

Disadvantages of buccal and sublingual routes of drug administration

- Due to the small size of the oral cavity, only very potent drugs can be effectively delivered. The buccal mucosa offers about 200 cm2 of area for drug absorption, i.e. about 10,000 times less than the duodenum.
- Difficulty in keeping the drug in the site, as well as the need for the patient to refrain from swallowing, talking, or drinking during administration so as not to affect the residence time in which the medication is in direct contact with the mucous membrane.
- Buccal and sublingual routes of administration do not apply to bitter or bad-tasting drugs since, in addition to patient discomfort, this type of formulation generates excessive production of saliva, which increases the risk of swallowing.

3. Rectal route

- Medications are sometimes ordered to be administered by rectal route. The rectal mucosa is capable of absorbing many soluble drugs into the circulation. Rectal medication may be in suppository form or in liquid form to be administered as a retention enema.
- Unlike the oral route, drugs with an irritant or unpalatable nature can be administered through the rectum. The rectal route can also be preferred when the patient has persistent vomiting or is unable to swallow. Also, this route can be used for systemic drug administration in addition to the local administration.

Advantages of the rectal route of drug administration

There are several scenarios in which the rectal route of drug administration may become the route of choice due to one of the following characteristics:

1. Applicable in cases of nausea, vomiting, and inability to swallow (unconscious patients), as well as in the presence of diseases of the upper gastrointestinal tract that affect oral drug absorption.
2. Suitable for formulations with unpleasant taste (a particularly important factor in children).
3. Allows achieving rapid systemic effects by giving a drug in a suitable solution (as an alternative to injection), with the additional advantage that such effect can be rapidly terminated in cases of toxicity or overdose. The absorption rate of the drug is not influenced by food or gastric emptying.
4. Part of the metabolism of both enteric and first-pass hepatic elimination is avoided, which may result in a significant increase in the bioavailability of extensively metabolized drugs (such as lidocaine).

Disadvantages of the rectal route of administration

Some drawbacks associated with rectal administration of pharmaceutical products include:

- The interruption of the absorption process by defecation, which can occur especially when the drug is irritant.
- Absorption can be highly irregular and incomplete.
- The reduced surface area may limit absorption, in the same way, that the low volume of rectal fluids can lead to incomplete dissolution of the drug.
- It is possible the degradation of certain drugs by microorganisms in the rectum.
  - Patient adherence may be a problem.

5. Transdermal route

The transdermal route is commonly referred to as "the patch" because the medication is contained in a patch that is absorbed through the skin. Drugs administered through this route must be highly lipophilic. Absorption via this route is slow but conducive to producing long-lasting effects. Special slow-release matrices in some transdermal patches can maintain steady drug concentrations that approach those of constant IV infusion. Transdermal patches also provide fewer absorption problems in the gastrointestinal tract that are commonly experienced by patients who take oral medications.

Drugs administered through this route include fentanyl patches for severe pain management, nitroglycerin transdermal patches used to prevent episodes of angina in people who have coronary artery disease, nicotine patches for cessation of smoking, etc.

6. Inhalational route/ pulmonary route

Drug delivery by inhalation is a common route, both for local and for systemic actions. This delivery route is particularly useful for the direct treatment of asthmatic problems, using both powder aerosols (e.g. salmeterol xinafoate) and pressurized metered-dose aerosols containing the drug in liquefied inert propellant (e.g. salbutamol sulphate inhaler).

Drugs may be inhaled as gases (e.g., nitrous oxide) and enter the bloodstream by diffusing across the alveolar membrane. This is the method of administration of volatile anaesthetics such as ether, halothane, and methoxyflurane.

The lungs provide an excellent surface for absorption when the drug is delivered in gaseous, aerosol mist or ultra-fine solid particle form. This results in rapid onset of action. Another advantage is that plasma concentration can be rapidly adjusted as well.

7. Injection routes/Parenteral Routes

This is the second commonest route of drug administration. They mainly involve introducing the drug in form of solution or suspension into the body at various sites and to varying depths using a syringe and needle. Thus administration involves the risk of infection, pain, and local irritation.

Injection routes of drug administration are usually employed where:

- Rapid effect is urgently needed in emergency situations;
- The patient is too ill or unconscious for an oral route to be employed;
- The drug is orally ineffective due to its being destroyed or not absorbed from the gut;
- An injection is the only way for the drug to reach its required site of action;

5. There is a need to maintain a steady blood level of a drug.

6. the most important factors or requirements in all injection routes are the surrounding tissue or site must be as clean as possible, and all instruments used must be clean and sterile. There are three commonly used injection routes: subcutaneous (SC), intramuscular (IM), and intravenous (IV). Other routes such as intra-arterial (IA), intrathecal (IT), intraperitoneal (IP), intravitreal etc., are used less frequently.

Injection routes

Definition

Subcutaneous (SC)

The administration beneath the skin; is hypodermic. Synonymous with the term subdermal or hypodermal.

Intramuscular (IM)

- ✓ Administration within a muscle.

Intradermal (ID)

- ✓ Administration within the dermis.

Intravenous (IV)

- ✓ Administration within or into a vein or veins.

Intra-arterial (IA)

- ✓ Administration within an artery or arteries.

Intrathecal (IT)

- ✓ Administration within the cerebrospinal fluid at any level of the cerebrospinal axis, including injection into the cerebral ventricles

Intraperitoneal (IP)

- ✓ Administration within the peritoneal cavity.

Intravitreal

- ✓ Administration within the vitreous body of the eye.

Pharmacokinetics

The term pharmacokinetics is derived from the ancient Greek words "pharmakon" and "kinetics", meaning "drug" and "putting in motion" respectively. It is one of the main branches of pharmacology and refers to the way that the body reacts to and affects a pharmaceutical substance in the body.

Or

Pharmacokinetics (PK) represents "what the body does to the drug"

From the moment that a drug enters the body, the body recognizes it and processes it uniquely, according to the individual characteristics of the drug. Pharmacokinetics is the study of how the body reacts to the presence of a drug. This information can be used to improve the administration and use of medicines.

There are four main components of pharmacokinetics: absorption, distribution, metabolism and excretion (ADME). These are used to explain the various characteristics of different drugs in the body.

Absorption

Absorption is the process in which a pharmaceutical substance enters the blood circulation in the body. The pharmacokinetic parameters for absorption include:

- The absorption rate constant: absorption rate/amount of drug remaining to be absorbed

- Bioavailability: the amount of drug absorbed / drug dose

- **Bioavailability:**

In pharmacology, bioavailability refers to the portion of an administered drug that reaches the systemic circulation through absorption. When a medication is given intravenously, its bioavailability is considered to be 100% by definition. However, when a medication is administered through non-intravenous routes, its bioavailability is generally lower due to factors like intestinal endothelium absorption and first-pass metabolism. Mathematically, bioavailability can be calculated as the ratio of the area under the plasma drug concentration curve versus time (AUC) for the extra vascular formulation to the AUC for the intravascular formulation. AUC is used for this purpose because it is directly proportional to the dose that has entered the systemic circulation.

The bioavailability of a drug is typically expressed as an average value, but to consider individual variability within a population, a deviation range is employed. This range accounts for differences among individuals, particularly those with poor absorption. In such cases, the bottom value of the deviation range is utilized to determine the real bioavailability and calculate the appropriate drug dose required for the individual to attain systemic concentrations similar to what would be achieved with the intravenous formulation. This approach ensures that the drug achieves the intended efficacy, even when the drug taker's absorption rate is unknown, except in situations where the drug has a narrow therapeutic window. In cases with a narrow therapeutic window, more precise dosing information is essential to avoid potential adverse effects.

Factors influencing bioavailability

The absolute bioavailability of a drug, when administered by an extravascular route, is usually less than one (i.e., F< 100%). Various physiological factors reduce the availability of drugs before they enter the systemic circulation. Whether a drug is taken with or without food will also affect absorption, other drugs taken concurrently may alter absorption and first-pass metabolism, intestinal motility alters the dissolution of the drug and may affect the degree of chemical degradation of the drug by intestinal microflora. Disease states affecting liver metabolism or gastrointestinal function will also have an effect.

Other factors may include, but are not limited to:

- ✓ Physical properties of the drug (hydrophobicity, pKa, solubility)
- ✓ The drug formulation (immediate release, excipients used, manufacturing methods, modified release – delayed-release, extended-release, sustained-release, etc.)
- ✓ Whether the formulation is administered in a fed or fasted state
- ✓ Gastric emptying rate
- ✓ Circadian differences

- ✓ Interactions with other drugs/foods:
- ✓ Interactions with other drugs (e.g., antacids, alcohol, nicotine)
- ✓ Interactions with other foods (e.g., grapefruit juice, pomelo, cranberry juice, brassica vegetables
- ✓ Transporters: Substrate of efflux transporters (e.g. P-glycoprotein)
- ✓ The health of the gastrointestinal tract

Enzyme induction/inhibition by other drugs/foods: Enzyme induction (increased rate of metabolism), e.g., Phenytoin induces CYP1A2, CYP2C9, CYP2C19, and CYP3A4. Enzyme inhibition (decreased rate of metabolism), e.g., grapefruit juice inhibits CYP3A → higher nifedipine concentrations

Individual variation in metabolic differences

Age: In general, drugs are metabolized more slowly in fetal, neonatal, and geriatric populations.

Phenotypic differences, enterohepatic circulation, diet, gender and Disease state

E.g., hepatic insufficiency, poor renal function

Each of these factors may vary from patient to patient (inter-individual variation), and indeed in the same patient over time (intra-individual variation). In clinical trials, inter-individual variation is a critical measurement used to assess the bioavailability differences from patient to patient in order to ensure predictable dosing.

Some of the key factors that can impact bioavailability include:

Route of Administration: Different routes of drug administration (oral, intravenous, intramuscular, etc.) can significantly affect how a drug is absorbed and its subsequent bioavailability.

Absorption Rate: The rate at which a drug is absorbed into the bloodstream from its site of administration can impact its bioavailability. Slow or incomplete absorption can lead to reduced bioavailability.

First-Pass Metabolism: When a drug is absorbed from the gastrointestinal tract, it may pass through the liver before entering the systemic circulation. If the drug undergoes significant metabolism during this "first pass" through the liver, its bioavailability can be reduced.

Chemical Properties: The physicochemical properties of a drug, such as its solubility, lipophilicity, and molecular size, can influence its ability to cross cell membranes and impact its bioavailability.

Food and Drug Interactions: Food intake, as well as interactions with other drugs or substances, can affect drug absorption and, consequently, bioavailability.

Gastric Emptying and Intestinal Transit: The rate at which the stomach empties and the drug moves through the intestines can influence drug absorption and bioavailability.

Drug Formulation: Different drug formulations (e.g., immediate-release, extended-release) can have varying rates of drug release and absorption, affecting bioavailability.

Disease Conditions: Certain medical conditions affecting the gastrointestinal tract or liver can alter drug absorption and bioavailability.

Age and Gender: Factors such as age and gender can sometimes influence drug metabolism and absorption, impacting bioavailability.

Genetic Variability: Genetic variations among individuals can lead to differences in drug metabolizing enzymes or drug transporters, affecting drug absorption and bioavailability.

First Pass Metabolism

The first-pass effect is a phenomenon in drug metabolism where the concentration of a drug, especially when administered orally, undergoes significant reduction before it enters the systemic circulation. This reduction occurs during the absorption process, primarily in the liver and gut wall. Several notable medications that experience a significant first-pass effect include Tofranil, morphine, propranolol, buprenorphine, diazepam, midazolam, pethidine, THC (psychoactive component of cannabis), alcohol (ethanol), cimetidine, lidocaine, and antipsychotic agents.

On the other hand, some drugs undergo increased potency due to the first-pass effect. For instance, the effect of THC, which is the most extensively studied active ingredient in cannabis, is enhanced by the conversion of a significant portion into 11-hydroxy-THC, resulting in greater efficiency compared to the original THC compound. This transformation contributes to the overall pharmacological effects experienced by individuals using cannabis.

First pass metabolism could occur within the liver (for propranolol, lidocaine, clomethiazole, and NTG) or within the gut (for penicillin G and insulin).

After a drug is ingested, it undergoes absorption into the bloodstream and enters the portal vascular system, which carries it to the liver before it circulates throughout the rest of the body. The liver plays a significant role in metabolizing many drugs, often to such an extent that only a small amount of the active drug is released from the liver to the systemic circulation. This initial passage through the liver, known as the "first pass," can significantly reduce the bioavailability of the drug as shown in Fig 1.

An example of a drug where first pass metabolism poses a complication and disadvantage is the antiviral medication Remdesivir. Due to its high liver metabolism, Remdesivir cannot be administered orally, as the entire dose would be trapped in the liver with little reaching the general circulation or the organs and cells affected by conditions like SARS-CoV-2. Therefore, Remdesivir is administered through intravenous (IV) infusion, bypassing the portal vascular system. However, significant liver extraction still occurs due to "second pass metabolism," whereby a fraction of blood travels through the portal vein and hepatocytes (liver cells).

By using the IV route, healthcare providers can ensure that enough of the drug reaches its target site and achieves the desired therapeutic effect without being excessively metabolized in the liver. This method optimizes the drug's bioavailability and effectiveness for treating the specific medical condition it is intended for.

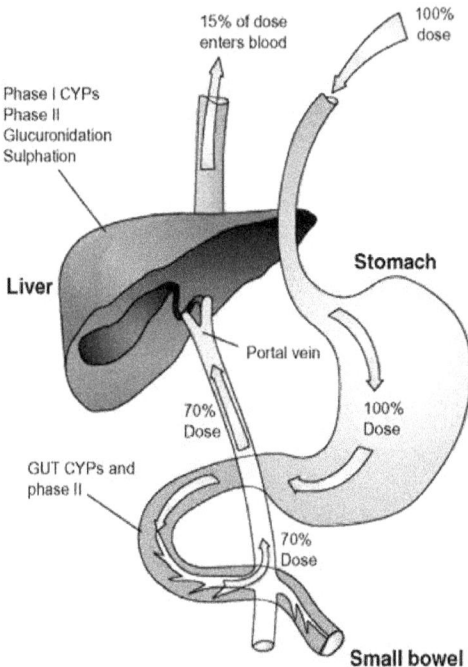

Fig.1 First Pass Metabolism

Excretion

Excretion is the process by which waste products, toxins, and other substances are removed from the body. It is an essential function of various organs and systems in the body, ensuring the elimination of metabolic by-products and substances that the body no longer needs or that might be harmful if retained.

The main organs involved in the excretion process are:

- Kidneys: The kidneys are responsible for filtering the blood and removing waste products, excess water, electrolytes, and toxins to form urine, which is then excreted from the body.
- Lungs: The lungs play a role in excretion by removing carbon dioxide and other gaseous waste products produced during cellular respiration.
- Skin: The skin helps in excretion through the process of sweating, which eliminates water, salts, and small amounts of waste products.
- Liver: The liver is involved in the excretion of certain waste products through bile secretion, which aids in the removal of substances processed by the liver, such as bilirubin and drugs.

- Intestines: The intestines are responsible for the elimination of undigested food and other waste materials as feces.

Excretion is a crucial aspect of maintaining the body's internal balance and preventing the buildup of harmful substances. Proper excretion ensures that waste products are efficiently eliminated, allowing the body to function effectively and remain healthy.

Pharmacokinetic Studies

Pharmacokinetic studies are a crucial part of pharmacology and clinical research that focus on understanding how drugs move within the body. These studies examine the processes of drug absorption, distribution, metabolism, and excretion, collectively known as ADME, over a period of time after drug administration. Pharmacokinetic studies help in determining the drug's behavior in the body, which is essential for designing safe and effective dosing regimens for patients. Some common types of pharmacokinetic studies include:

- **Absorption Studies:** These studies investigate how drugs are absorbed into the bloodstream after administration through different routes, such as oral, intravenous, intramuscular, or subcutaneous routes.
- **Distribution Studies:** These studies examine how drugs are distributed to various tissues and organs in the body after entering the bloodstream. They can determine the drug's volume of distribution and tissue penetration.
- **Metabolism Studies:** These studies focus on understanding how drugs are metabolized or biotransformed in the body, typically in the liver, into different metabolites that may be active or inactive.
- **Excretion Studies**: These studies analyze the elimination of drugs and their metabolites from the body, often through urine, feces, or exhalation.
- **Plasma Concentration-Time Profiling:** Pharmacokinetic studies involve measuring the concentration of a drug in the bloodstream over time, which helps to calculate important parameters like half-life, clearance, and area under the plasma concentration-time curve (AUC).
- **Drug-Drug Interaction Studies**: These studies assess how one drug may affect the pharmacokinetics of another drug when administered together, potentially leading to altered efficacy or safety profiles.

➤ **Population Pharmacokinetic Studies**: These studies involve analyzing pharmacokinetic data from a group of patients to identify any potential variations based on age, gender, ethnicity, or other factors.

Pharmacokinetic studies are fundamental in the drug development process, ensuring that medications are administered safely and effectively to patients. They also help healthcare professionals in selecting appropriate dosing regimens for individuals based on their unique pharmacokinetic characteristics.

Half-Life of a Drug

The elimination half-life of a drug could be a pharmacokinetic parameter that's outlined because the time it takes for the concentration of the drug within the plasma or the overall quantity within the body to be reduced by five hundredth. In different words, once one half-life, the concentration of the drug within the body are going to be half the beginning dose. With every extra half-life, proportionately less of the drug is eliminated. However, the time needed for the drug to achieve half the initial concentration remains constant. In general, the result of the drug is taken into account to own a negligible therapeutic result once four half-lives, that's once solely six.25% of the initial dose remains within the body. Illustrative example

If a one hundred weight unit (mg) dose of associate degree blood vessel drug with a half-life of quarter-hour is run, the subsequent would be true:

1. 15 minutes once the drug administration, fifty mg of the drug remains within the body.
2. 30 minutes once the drug administration, twenty five mg of the drug remains within the body.
3. 45 minutes once the drug administration, 12.5 mg of the drug remains within the body.
4. 1 hour once the drug administration, 6.25 mg of the drug remains within the body.
5. hours once the drug administration, 0.39 mg of the drug remains within the body.

Related terms

Several different terms square measure closely associated with the drug half-life, including:

The elimination rate constant (λ): This describes the speed of drug elimination from the body as a fraction. This worth is constant in first-order dynamics and freelance of drug concentration.

Apparent half-life: In some circumstances, like controlled-release formulations, the decline within the concentration of the drug isn't exclusively hooked in to elimination, however conjointly on the speed of absorption and distribution that influences the discovered half-life.

Clinical uses

The elimination half-life could be a helpful pharmacokinetic parameter, because it provides associate degree correct indication of the length of your time that the result of the drug persists in a personal.

Moreover, the elimination half-life may also show if associate degree accumulation of the drug is probably going to occur with a multiple dosing plan. This can be useful once it involves deciding the suitable dose and frequency of a prescribed drug.

Along with different pharmacokinetic information and values concerning the individual patient, the half-life will facilitate health practitioners to estimate the speed at that a drug are going to be eliminated from the body, additionally as what proportion can stay once a given time. From this data, acceptable choices are created on a way to promote patient health outcomes.

1. Ligand-gated ion channels

Ligand-gated ion channels, also known as ionotropic receptors, are integral membrane proteins that play a crucial role in the transmission of signals in the nervous system and other tissues. These receptors are involved in fast synaptic transmission and allow ions to pass through a channel when they are bound to a specific ligand, such as a neurotransmitter or hormone. This ligand binding induces a conformational change in the receptor, resulting in the opening or closing of an ion channel. Fig. 2 Here are some key characteristics of ligand-gated ion channels:

Ligand Binding: Ligand-gated ion channels are activated when a specific ligand, such as a neurotransmitter like glutamate, GABA, or acetylcholine, binds to the receptor. The binding site is often on the extracellular side of the receptor.

Fast Signaling: These channels mediate rapid and direct responses to neurotransmitters, allowing for the fast transmission of signals between nerve cells (neurons) and at neuromuscular junctions.

Ion Selectivity: Ligand-gated ion channels are often selective for specific ions, such as sodium (Na^+), potassium (K^+), calcium (Ca^{2+}), or chloride (Cl^-). The ion permeability of the channel depends on the specific receptor.

Channel Gating: When the ligand binds to the receptor, it induces a conformational change that opens or closes an ion channel within the receptor's structure. This allows ions to flow through the membrane.

Neurotransmitter Release: After the ion channel opens, the movement of ions across the cell membrane leads to changes in the membrane potential, which can generate electrical signals. This, in turn, can trigger the release of neurotransmitters from the neuron's presynaptic terminal.

Examples:

- *Nicotinic Acetylcholine Receptors:* Found at the neuromuscular junction and in the central nervous system, they are activated by acetylcholine.
- *Glutamate Receptors:* Include AMPA receptors, NMDA receptors, and kainate receptors, which are involved in excitatory synaptic transmission.
- *GABA Receptors*: Mediate inhibitory synaptic transmission and include GABAA and GABAB receptors.
- *Serotonin (5-HT3) Receptors*: Activated by serotonin and play a role in mood regulation and other functions.

Ligand-gated ion channels are essential for the rapid and precise communication between neurons in the nervous system. Dysregulation of these receptors can have profound effects on brain function and can contribute to various neurological and psychiatric disorders.

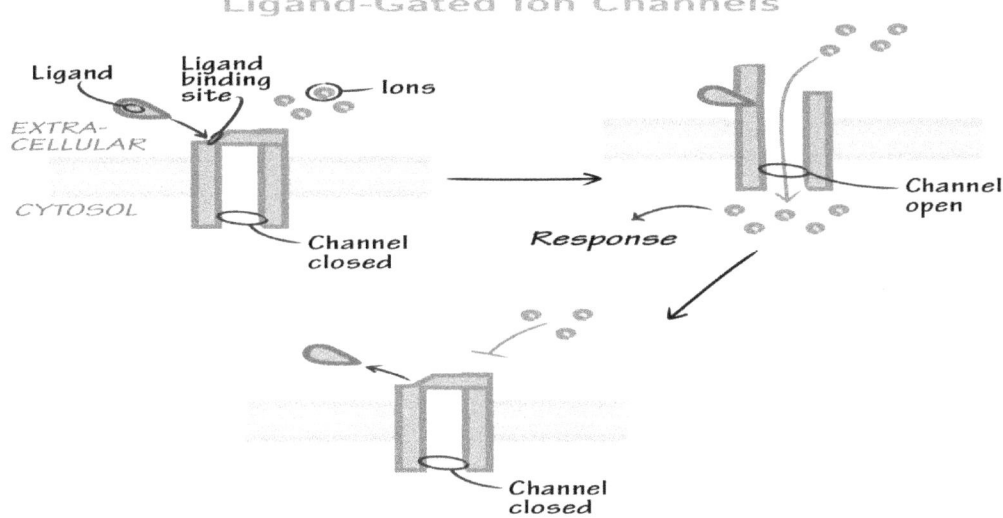

Fig.2 Ligand-gated ion channel synaptic transmission

2. GPCR

G protein-coupled receptors (GPCRs), also known as **seven-(pass)-transmembrane domain receptors**, **7TM receptors**, **heptahelical receptors**, **serpentine receptors**, and **G protein-linked receptors (GPLR)**, form a large group of evolutionarily-related proteins that are cell surface receptors that detect molecules outside the cell and activate cellular responses. Coupling with G proteins, they are called seven-transmembrane receptors because they pass through the cell membrane seven times. Ligands can bind either to extracellular N-terminus and loops (e.g. glutamate receptors) or to the binding site within transmembrane helices (Rhodopsin-like family). They are all activated by agonists although a spontaneous auto-activation of an empty receptor can also be observed.

G protein-coupled receptors are found only in eukaryotes, including yeast, choanoflagellates and animals. The ligands that bind and activate these receptors include light-sensitive compounds, odors, pheromones, hormones, and neurotransmitters, and vary in size from small molecules to peptides to large proteins. G protein-coupled receptors are involved in many diseases.

Type 2: Metabotropic receptors (G protein-coupled receptors) – This is the largest receptor family, containing receptors for a variety of hormones and slow transmitters such as dopamine and metabotropic glutamate. They are made up of seven alpha helices that run across the membrane. Extracellular and intracellular domains are formed by the loops connecting the alpha helices. Larger peptide ligands often bind in the extracellular domain, whereas smaller non-peptide ligands typically bind between the seven alpha helices and one extracellular loop. G proteins connect the aforementioned receptors to several intracellular effector systems. G proteins are heterotrimers consisting of three subunits: (alpha), (beta), and (gamma) (gamma). The three subunits interact in the inactive state, and the -subunit binds GDP. The activation of G proteins results in a conformational shift. Furthermore, the three subunits, α, β, and γ have additional four main classes based on their primary sequence. These include G_s, G_i, G_q and G_{12}.

There are two principal signal transduction pathways involving the G protein-coupled receptors:

- *the cAMP signal pathway and*

- *the phosphatidylinositol signal pathway.*

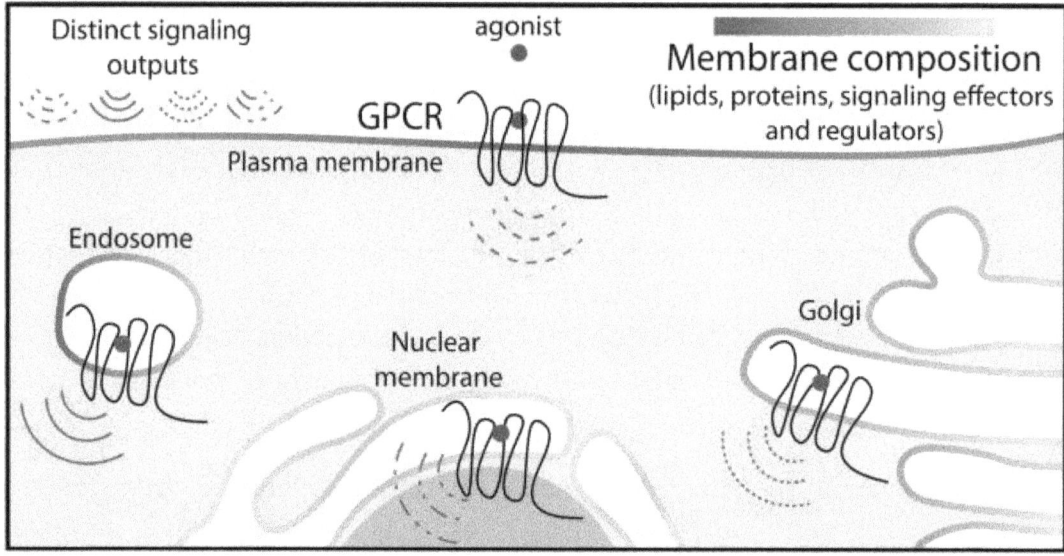

Fig.3 G protein-coupled receptors (GPCRs), transmembrane domain receptors, 7TM receptors, heptahelical receptors, serpentine receptors, and G protein-linked receptors (GPLR)

When a ligand binds to a GPCR, it causes the GPCR to alter conformation, allowing it to function as a guanine nucleotide exchange factor (GEF). By exchanging the

GDP linked to the G protein for GTP, the GPCR can then activate a related G protein. Depending on the subunit type (Gs, Gi/o, Gq/11, G12/13), the G protein's subunit, together with the bound GTP, can subsequently separate from the and subunits to alter intracellular signalling proteins or target functional proteins directly.

GPCRs are a popular drug target, with 108 members of this family being targeted by nearly 34% of all FDA-approved medicines. As of 2018, the global market for these medications is anticipated to be over 180 billion dollars. GPCRs are thought to be targets for about half of all drugs currently on the market, owing to their role in signalling pathways linked to a variety of diseases, including mental, metabolic, including endocrinological disorders, immunological, including viral infections, cardiovascular, inflammatory, senses, and cancer. Another dynamically emerging topic of pharmacological study is the long-known relationship between GPCRs and a variety of endogenous and exogenous drugs, which results in analgesia, for example.

3. Enzyme-linked hormone receptors

Hormone receptors are specialized proteins that specifically bind to particular hormones, forming hormone-receptor complexes. These receptors are divided into two categories: transmembrane receptors, found on the cell surface, and intracellular or nuclear receptors, located within the cytoplasm or nucleus. Transmembrane receptors respond to peptide hormones, while intracellular receptors interact with lipid-soluble hormones like steroid hormones. When hormones bind to their respective receptors, they activate signaling pathways, leading to various cellular responses and changes in the body. These interactions are crucial for maintaining homeostasis and mediating the effects of hormones in the body. Understanding hormone-receptor interactions is essential for developing targeted therapies and managing hormonal conditions.

Type 3: Kinase-linked and related receptors, also known as "Receptor tyrosine kinases" (RTKs) and "Enzyme-linked receptors," are cell surface receptors characterized by their structure. They consist of an extracellular domain for ligand binding, an intracellular domain with enzymatic activity, and are connected by a single transmembrane alpha helix. When their specific ligand binds to the extracellular domain, these receptors undergo a conformational change, leading to the activation of their enzymatic activity. This activation triggers intracellular signaling cascades that regulate various cellular processes, including growth, differentiation, and survival. RTKs and enzyme-linked receptors are crucial for normal growth and development, and their dysregulation is associated with various diseases, making them important targets for biomedical research and drug development. The insulin receptor is an example of this type of receptor..

Agonist vs Antagonist

- *(Full) agonists* can activate the receptor and result in a strong biological response. The natural endogenous ligand with the greatest efficacy for a given receptor is by definition a full agonist (100% efficacy).

- *Partial agonists* do not activate receptors with maximal efficacy, even with maximal binding, causing partial responses compared to those of full agonists (efficacy between 0 and 100%).

- *Antagonists* attach to receptors but do not make them active. This inhibits the binding of agonists and inverse agonists, resulting in a receptor blockade. Competitive (or reversible) antagonists compete with the agonist for receptor binding, whereas irreversible antagonists establish covalent bonds (or exceptionally high-affinity non-covalent bonds) with the receptor and fully block it. One example of an irreversible antagonist is the proton pump inhibitor omeprazole. Only the production of new receptors can counteract the consequences of irreversible antagonistism.

- *Inverse agonists* reduce the activity of receptors by inhibiting their constitutive activity (negative efficacy).

- *Allosteric modulators*: They bind to specific allosteric binding sites on the receptor rather than the agonist binding site, and so change the function of the agonist. Benzodiazepines (BZDs), for example, bind to the GABAA receptor's BZD site and enhance the impact of endogenous GABA.

- **Note** that the idea of receptor agonism and antagonism only refers to the interaction between receptors and ligands and not to their biological effects.

Some examples of ionotropic (LGIC) and metabotropic (specifically, GPCRs) receptors are shown in the table 1 below. The chief neurotransmitters are glutamate and GABA; other neurotransmitters are neuromodulatory. This list is by no means exhaustive.

Neurotransmitter	Ionotropic Receptors (LGIC)	Metabotropic Receptors (GPCRs)
Glutamate	NMDA receptor	Glutamate receptors: mGluR1 to mGluR8
	AMPA receptor	
	Kainate receptor	
GABA	GABAA receptor	GABAB receptor
Other Neuromodulatory Neurotransmitters	Acetylcholine: Nicotinic acetylcholine receptors (nAChRs) Muscarinic acetylcholine receptors (mAChRs)	Dopamine: D1 receptor Dopamine: D2 receptor Serotonin: 5-HT1A receptor
	Adenosine: Adenosine receptors (A1, A2A, A2B, A3)	Serotonin: 5-HT2A receptor
	Histamine: Histamine receptors (H1, H2, H3, H4)	

Table 1 examples of ionotropic (LGIC) and metabotropic (specifically, GPCRs) receptors

DRUG USED IN CARDIOLOGY HYPERTENSION AND RELATED PATHOLOGIES

Classification and mechanism of action,

Centrally acting medication is a type of medication that acts on the central nervous system (Clonidine and methyldopa), Classification of vasodilators and metal channel blockers, as well as medications affecting the angiotonin system's proteolytic enzyme. Anti-anginous medications; central nervous system (Clonidine and methyldopa),

categorization of drugs that impact the proteolytic enzyme of the angiotensin system, including calcium channel blockers and vasodilators. Drugs that reduce inflammation; medicine that operates on the central nervous system is referred to as centrally acting medicine (methyldopa and clonidine) categorization of drugs that influence the proteolytic enzyme of the angiotonin system, including metal channel blockers and vasodilators. anti-inflammatory drugs;

- **Classification and medicine of anti -anginal medication**.

Anti-arrhythmic drugs; Classification and mechanism of action, medicine of Quinidex (An early kind metallic element channel blocker), Salient options of different anti-arrhythmic medication,

Drugs used for medical care of symptom internal organ failure (CCF); Classification and mechanism of action of medication used for CCF, medicine of digitalis,

Salient options of different medication employed in CCF. medication employed in treatment of hyperlipidaemias;

Classification and mechanism of action of anti- hyperlipidaemics, medicine of lipid- lowering medication (A early sort of HMG CoA enzyme inhibitor),

- **Salient options of different anti- hyperlipidaemic agents.**

a) **Anti- hypertensive agents:**

Classification and mechanism of action Blood pressure- it's the lateral pressure exerted by the blood on its wall. flow (CO) determines the heartbeat BP, whereas peripheral resistance (PR) determines the beat BP. traditional BP 120/80 mmHg Purpose of HT treatment- it's not solely to lower the BP, however to shield the target organs-heart, brain, eyes, and kidneys. These organs ar broken if HT isn't properly controlled.

BLOOD PRESSURE CATEGORY	SYSTOLIC mm Hg (upper number)		DIASTOLIC mm Hg (lower number)
NORMAL	LESS THAN 120	and	LESS THAN 80
ELEVATED	120 – 129	and	LESS THAN 80
HIGH BLOOD PRESSURE (HYPERTENSION) STAGE 1	130 – 139	or	80 – 89
HIGH BLOOD PRESSURE (HYPERTENSION) STAGE 2	140 OR HIGHER	or	90 OR HIGHER
HYPERTENSIVE CRISIS (consult your doctor immediately)	HIGHER THAN 180	and/or	HIGHER THAN 120

Classification of medicine

1. Centrally acting medicine - antihypertensive drug, α antihypertensive drug

2. Ganglion blockers- a-Competitive neural structure blockers: Trimetaphan, Tetraethylammonium (TEA), Mecamylamine, and Pempidine.

B. Non competitive neural structure blockers: Hexamethoneum

3. Adrenergic vegetative cell blockers- Sandril, guanethidine.

4. α blockers- α1 and α2 blockers- anit-impotence drug, and phenoxybenzamine. Specific α1 blockers- alpha-adrenergic blocker, terazosin, doxazosin.

5. β blockers- Non selective β blockers- Propranolol, β1 blockers- beta blocker, Metoprolol,

6. Calcium channel blockers (CCB) – Verapamil, diltiazem, nifedipine, amlodipine.

7. ACE inhibitors- lisinopril, enalapril, ramipril, benazepril.

8. Angiotensin receptor Blocker- losartan, telmisartan, valasertan, candesartan.

9. Direct acting vasodilators- minoxidil, sodium nitroprusside

10. Mineralocorticoid antagonist- Spironolactone

11. Diuretics- Thiazides and loop diuretics- furosemide.

Mechanism of actions of medicine medicine

1. Centrally acting drugs- antihypertensive drug, α antihypertensive drug Clonidine-

It acts on α2 receptors (auto-receptors) placed within the constriction center of the brain. The presynaptic membranes of the adrenergic nerve endings of the constriction center have α2 receptors. Upon stimulation the discharged adrenaline/Nor-adrenaline additionally binds to those receptors. These receptors belong to the Gi variety of G supermolecule coupled receptors. The activation of α2 receptors causes activation of K+ channel, closure of Ca2+ channel. This results in hyperpolarization (IPSP). This decreases the secretion of nor-adrenaline and leading to vasodilatation (due to belittled interaction between nor-adrenaline with alpha receptors placed on the vascular swish muscles). This decreases peripheral resistance within the blood vessels and heartbeat BP. The belittled sympathetic activity additionally decreases force of contraction of the guts and flow rate. This decreases beat B.P. so antihypertensive drug decreases each heartbeat and blood pressure. Antihypertensive drug –It is a medicinal drug and is that the L-isomer of alpha-methyldopa. Its brand is antihypertensive drug. It's a twin mechanism of action

1. It acts by inhibiting the catalyst dihydroxyphenylalanine enzyme (it converts levodopa to dopamine). This ends up in belittled formation of noradrenaline/adrenaline. This decreases B.P

2. Dopastat Dopastat converts α methyl radical-dopa to methyl nor-adrenaline within the conjugation vesicles of the sympathetic nerves. The discharged methyl radical nor-adrenaline acts as false neurotransmitters for the alpha receptors gift on the blood vessels. This interaction ends up in vasodilatation and reduces the **BP.**

2. Neural structure blockersa-Competitive neural structure blockers: Trimetaphan, Tetraethylammonium (TEA), Mecamylamine, and Pempidine.

b. Non competitive neural structure blockers: Hexamethoneum Ganglionic blockers block each sympathetic and parasympathetic ganglia. These medicine square measure potent medicine medicine however their use is proscribed to short term treatment of high blood pressure related to dissecting cardiovascular disease of artery (when AN artery enclose the artery weakens, the wall abnormally expands or bulges as blood is wired through it, inflicting AN arterial blood vessel aneurysm) and within the production of controlled cardiovascular disease throughout surgery. three Ganglionic blockers act by interference the Nn receptors found within the sympathetic and parasympathetic ganglia. The neurotransmitter is that the agonist for the Nn receptors having each affinity and intrinsic activity. however ganglionic blockers have solely affinity. They bind to the binding web site placed within the 2 alpha subunits of the Nn receptors. thanks to blockage the nicotinic receptors no conformational modification within the pore size within the receptors. thus the metallic element particle fails to have the receptors. This initiates the repressive post conjugation potential (IPSP) and also the unharness of neurotransmitters (adrenaline/NA, acetylcholine) decreases. The belittled unharness of adrenaline/NA neurotransmitters causes medicine result.

3. Adrenergic vegetative cell blockers- Sandril, guanethidine Reserpine- it's AN organic compound obtained from snakewood. It irreversibly blocks the sac amine transporter (VMAT). The VMAT may be a transport supermolecule integrated into the membrane of conjugation vesicles of presynaptic neurons. VMAT square measure answerable for the uptake of cytosolic monoamines (eg Dopastat, nor-adrenaline, histamine, serotonin, etc) into vesicles in monoaminergic neurons. Unprotected neurotransmitters (nor-adrenaline and dopamine) square measure metabolized by MAO and COMT within the protoplasm. This results in belittled secretion of monoamine neurotransmitter and belittled BP. Its use is restricted in high blood pressure thanks to its depletion of neurochemical result. Guanethidine- it's AN medicinal drug that reduces the discharge of nor-adrenaline. Guanethidine is transported across the sympathetic nerve membrane (re uptake mechanism) the same as nor-adrenaline. Within the nerve terminal guanethidine is focused within the conjugation vesicles, wherever it replaces the nor-adrenaline. This results in a gradual depletion of nor-adrenaline stores within the nerve endings. This results in a gradual depletion of vasoconstrictive. This inhibits the discharge of nor-adrenaline and reduces the BP. it's prohibited in most of the country. however in some countries (eg.UK), it's used for the fast management of BP in hypertensive emergency

4. α blockers- α1 and α2 blockers- Phentolamine, and phenoxybenzamine. They blocks both α1 and α2 receptors. α2 blockage increases the sympathetic flow-> increase in HR. Hence they are not preferred except in pheochromocytoma. Specific α1 blockers- Prazosin, terazosin, doxazosin. They are selective α1 blockers. α1 stimulation produces vasoconstriction. Blockage of these receptors result in vasodilatation-> decrease in PR-> fall in BP. Vasodilatation occurs in both arteries and veins. Arterial dilatation causes decrease in PR, this decrease diastolic BP. Venodilatation decreases the venous return and cause decrease in CO and decrease in systolic BP. They also decrease TG, LDL and increase HDL.

5. β blockers- Non selective β blockers- Propranolol, β1 blockers- atenolol, Metoprolol,

MOA: .β1 receptors are located in the heart (pace maker cells and myocardial cells). β1 receptors belongs to Gs type of G protein coupled receptors. Adrenaline/NA are the agonist for these receptors. Propranalol, atenolol or Metoprolol are the antagonists for these receptors as they have only affinity with these receptors. The blockage of β1 receptors in the pacemaker cells by these drugs causes decrease in HR. The blockage in the myocardial cells decreases the force of heart contraction. This decreases the cardiac output. The decreased CO leads to decreased systolic BP.

Initially peripheral resistance (PR) increased, then normal and later there is marked decrease in the PR. This decreases the diastolic BP also. The beta blockers also block the β1 receptors located in the juxta-glomerular cells of the nephrons. The blockage by beta blockers decreases renin secretion and rennin decreases the BP through rennin-angiotension-aldosterone pathway.

6. Calcium channel blockers (CCB) - Verapamil, diltiazem, nifedipine, amlodipine. Mechanisms1.In cardiac cells troponin-tropomycin system prevents the interaction between actin and myosin. The calcium binding site present in the troponin. When adrenaline/NA binds to β2 (Gs) receptors, adenylyl cyclise (AC) gets activated. Activated AC stimulates the synthesis of cAMP (second messenger). The cAMP causes activation of cellular protein- protein kinase

1. The activated PKC causes the phosphorylation of other proteins like calcium channels. This increases the calcium concentration within the cell. These calcium ions bind to binding sites present in the troponin molecules. This disturbs the tropomycin-toponin system. This leads to the interaction between actin-myosin, and causes muscle contraction. In presence calcium channel blockers these calcium channels get blocked. This causes muscle relaxation. This reduces the heart contraction and cardiac output. This decreases systolic pressure (sBP).

2. In vascular smooth muscle cells- When sympathetic nerves get stimulated vasoconstriction takes place. The released adrenaline/NA binds to α1 receptors (Gq type) and stimulates the PLC. This leads to the formation of IP3 and DAG. These second messengers lead to increased intracellular concentration of calcium. Calcium combines with calmodulin to form Ca^{2+} - CaM complex, which activates MLCK. Activated MLCK phosphorylates myosin LC-> myosin LC- (P). This leads to vascular smooth muscle contraction (vasoconstriction). When calcium channels are blocked, there is; decreased entry of Ca^{2+} into the cell, decreased release of Ca^{2+} from SR, reduction in intracellular Ca^{2+}. Hence vasodilatation takes place. This decreases peripheral resistance (PR) and decreases diastolic BP. Thus calcium channel blockers reduce both systolic and diastolic B.P.

7. Angiotensin converting enzyme inhibitors- (ACE inhibitors)- Captopril, lisinopril, enalapril, ramipril, benazepril.

ACE inhibitors are the enzyme which inhibits the formation of angiotensin II. Fig.4 ACE is a membrane bound, zinc dependent dipeptidase that catalyzes the conversion of the decapeptide angiotensin I to the potent vasopressor octa-peptide angiotensin II by removing the two Cterminal amino acids. ACE is well known enzyme that regulates the BP through renninangiotensin-aldosterone pathway. Angiotensin II increases the BP by three waysa. Stimulates adrenal cortex. This increases the release of aldosterone. In the kidney aldosterone increases the tubular re-absorption of sodium and water. This increases blood volume and BP.

b. **Angiotensin II** also stimulates posterior pituitary gland. This increases the release of antidiuretic hormone (ADH). This hormone also increases the increases the tubular re-absorption of sodium and water. This increases blood volume and BP.

c. **Angiotensin II** directing act on the Angiotensin II receptors located on the vascular smooth muscles. This leads to vasoconstriction and increase in BP. ACE inhibitors act by inhibiting the ACE. This decreases the formation of angiotensin II and BP.

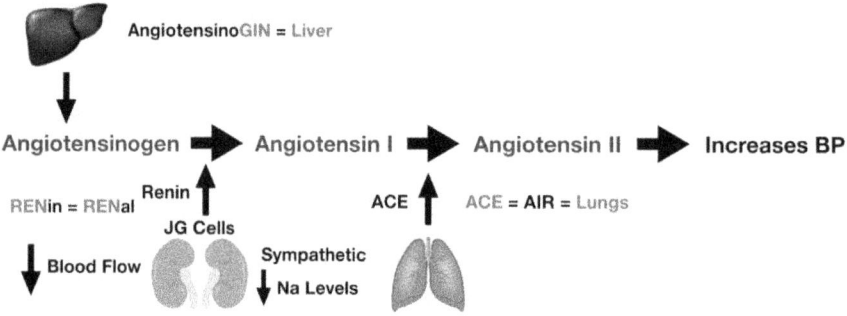

Fig.4 Angiotensin converting enzyme inhibitors- (ACE inhibitors) Mechanism of action

8. Angiotensin receptor antagonist- losartan, telmisartan, valasartan, candesartan. The angiotensin receptors (A1) are found in the heart, blood vessels, kidney, adrenal cortex, lung and brain. Its ligand is angiotension II. A1 receptors belong to G protein coupled receptors (Gq). When Angiotensin II binds to AI receptors the PLC get activated and the IP3 and DAG (second messengers) increase the calcium concentration within the cell. The calcium binds to Calcalmodulin complex. This complex stimulates the MLCK and causes phosphorylation of MLC to MLC-P. This causes vasoconstriction and increase of BP. Angiotensin receptor antagonists act by blocking the A1 receptors. This causes vasodilatation and decrease of BP. 5

9. Direct acting vasodilators- Hydralazine, minoxidil, Sodium nitropresside, Hydralazine is a direct acting smooth muscle relaxant used to treat hypertension by acting as a vasodilator primarily in arteries and arterioles. This decreases the peripheral resistance and BP. The exact mechanism of hydralazide is unknown. But it uses NO released from endothelium of the blood vessels for initiating its vasodilatory effect. Minoxidil- Minoxidil is an antihypertensive vasodilator medication. It also slows or stops hair loss. At present it is available OTC for the treatment of alopecia. Minoxidil is a prodrug activated by sulfation (addition of sulphate group) via the sulfotransferase. Minoxidil is a potassium channel opener, causing hyperpolarization of cell membranes and causes vasodilation. Na nitropresside is an inorganic compound. In the blood circulation Na nitropresside breaks to form NO. The NO diffuses into smooth muscle cell of blood vessel. NO activates guanylate cyclise and increases the concentration of cGMP. The cGMP activates protein kinase G. The activated protein kinase activates phosphatases, which inactivates myosin light chains by dephophorylation (MLC-P - MLC). This causes vasodilatation and reduces the BP.

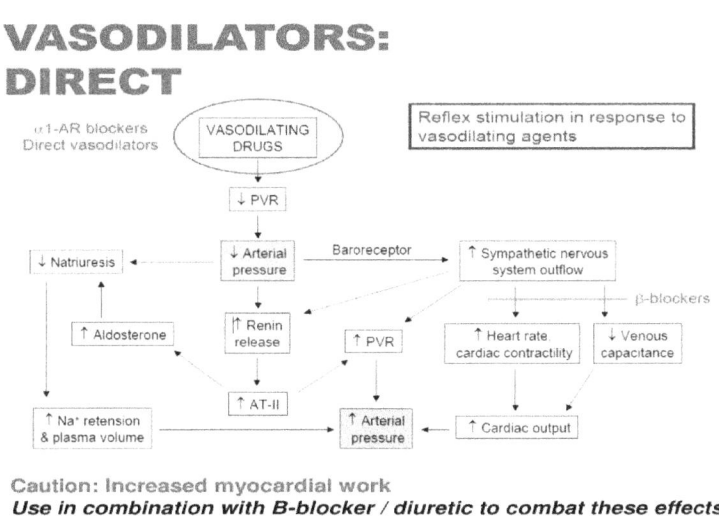

Fig.5 Direct acting vasodilators

10. Mineralocorticoid antagonist- eg-Spironolactone Spironolactone functions as a selective inhibitor of mineralocorticoids, primarily by competing for binding with receptors located at the aldosterone-sensitive sodium-potassium exchange site in the distal convoluted tubules. This results in increased excretion of sodium and water while maintaining potassium levels. Essentially, spironolactone serves a dual purpose as both a diuretic and an anti-hypertensive medication.

11. Diuretics- Thiazide diuretics are commonly used to manage high blood pressure and edema, which can result from conditions like heart, liver, or kidney disease. Thiazides are considered cost-effective medications. They function by inhibiting the sodium-chloride co-transporters in the distal convoluted tubules (DCT). These co-transporters are expressed on the cells in the DCT, leading to the reabsorption of sodium and chloride ions into the bloodstream. Thiazide diuretics work by blocking these co-transporters, reducing the reabsorption of sodium ions and thereby lowering blood pressure.

On the other hand, loop diuretics, such as furosemide (Frusemide), block the sodium-potassium-chloride co-transporters in the thick ascending limb of the loop of Henle, decreasing the reabsorption of sodium and chloride ions.

In addition to diuretics, centrally acting antihypertensive drugs, like Clonidine and methyldopa, have their own mechanism of action. Clonidine hydrochloride (Catapres) is derived from imidazoline and acts as a centrally acting alpha-2 receptor agonist, effectively lowering blood pressure.

Mechanism- Clonidine exerts its effects by acting on alpha-2 receptors, specifically the auto-receptors located in the brain's vasodilation center. These alpha-2 receptors are present on the presynaptic membranes of adrenergic nerve endings in the vasodilation center. When these receptors are stimulated, they bind to both freely circulating adrenaline and noradrenaline. These receptors belong to the Gi class of G-protein coupled receptors.

Activation of alpha-2 receptors leads to the activation of potassium (K+) channels and the closure of calcium (Ca2+) channels. This, in turn, causes hyperpolarization, resulting in inhibitory postsynaptic potentials (IPSP). This process reduces the release of noradrenaline, leading to vasodilation. Vasodilation occurs because there is less interaction between noradrenaline and the alpha receptors found on the smooth muscles of blood vessels. As a result, peripheral resistance in the blood vessels decreases, lowering both systolic and diastolic blood pressure. Furthermore, reduced sympathetic activity also leads to a decrease in the force of the heart's contractions and heart rate, further contributing to the decrease in blood pressure. Therefore, clonidine has a dual effect on lowering both systolic and diastolic blood pressure.m Metabolism-wise, clonidine undergoes liver metabolism through various cytochrome P450 enzymes, yielding four metabolites. However, only one of these metabolites, known as 4-norclonidine, is identified. Both this metabolite and the unaltered drug (clonidine) are eliminated from the body through urine.

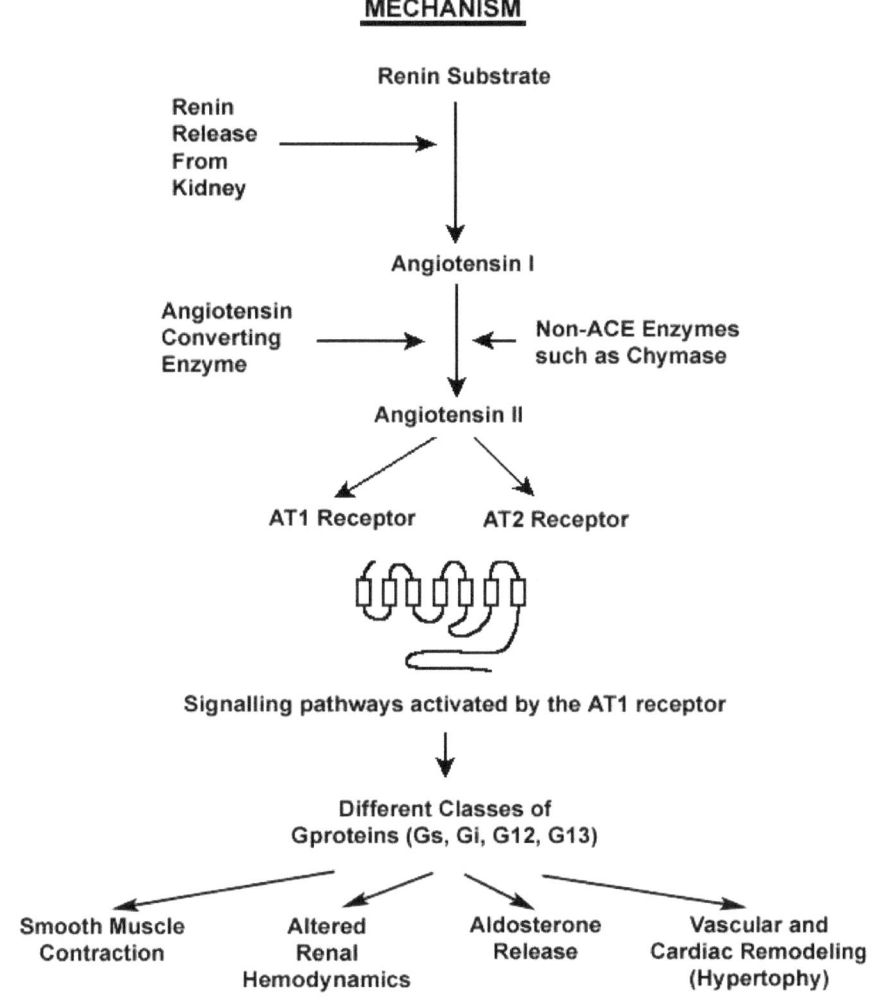

ADRs (Adverse Drug Reaction)- 6

1. Drowsiness, sedation, constipation, dryness of mouth, nose, and eyes.

2. Impotence, salt and water retention, bradycardia

3. Postural hypotension (drop in BP due to change in body position). Fluid retention and edema is also a problem with chronic therapy, therefore, concurrent therapy with a diuretic is necessary. Sudden discontinuation of clonidine can lead to rebound hypertension, which is due to excessive sympathetic activity.

Uses-

1. It is used to treat moderate and severe hypertension.

2. for the diagnosis and treatment of Pheochromocytoma-.

3. Used for the treatment of diarrhoea in diabetic patients.

4. Prophylaxis of migraine.

5. Used in attention deficit hyperactivity disorder (ADHD). **Contraindications**- In pregnancy, lactating women.

Drug interactions- If clonidine is given along with alcohol may cause sedation, poor judgement, slowdown of reflexes. Preparations- Clonidine HCl tablets, injection, transdermal patches. A methyl-dopa (aldomet) –It is a centrally acting antihypertensive drug.

Mechanism of Action-

It is an antihypertensive drug and is the L-isomer of alpha-methyldopa. Its brand name is aldomet. It has a dual mechanism of action

1. It acts by inhibiting the enzyme DOPA decarboxylase (it converts L-DOPA to dopamine). This results in decreased formation of noradrenaline/adrenaline. This decreases B.P

2. Dopamine β-hydroxylase converts α methyl-dopa to methyl nor-adrenaline in the synaptic vesicles of the sympathetic nerves. The released methyl nor-adrenaline acts as false neurotransmitters for the alpha receptors present on the blood vessels. This interaction results in vasodilatation and decreases the BP. Pharmacokinetics-

Methyldopa exhibits variable absorption from the gastrointestinal tract. It is metabolized in the liver and the intestine and is excreted in urine. The important metabolites are methyl alpha methyldopa, methyl alpha dopamine, alpha methyldopa sulphate, alpha methyl dopamine. ADRs- Sedation, lethargy, cognitive and memory impairment. Dryness of mouth, nasal stiffness, headache, fluid retention, weight gain, sexual dysfunction (libido, impotence), postural hypotension.

Uses-

It is used in moderate to severe hypertension in combination with a diuretic. It is safe during pregnancy. It is not indicated in pheochromocytoma. It is indicated in gestational hypertension (pregnancy induced hypertension) and in pre-eclampsia (it is a disorder in pregnancy characterized by high blood pressure and a large amount of protein in the urine. Usually it occurs at third trimester of pregnancy). Marketed Prep- Methyl dopa-125,250,500 mg tabs, 30mg/ml inj.

c. **Classification of vasodilators including calcium channel blockers**, Pharmacology of drugs affecting Renin Angiotensin system. Classification of vasodilators used in hypertension

1. Calcium channel blockers (CCB) - Verapamil, diltiazem, nifedipine, amlodipine.

2.ACE- inhibitors- Captopril, lisinopril, enalapril, ramipril, benazepril 3.Angiotensin receptor antagonist- Saralasin, losartan, telmisertan, valasertan, candesertan.

4.Direct acting vasodilators- Hydralazine, minoxidil, Na nitropressidePharmacology of drugs affecting Renin Angiotensin system. Pharmacology of ACE- inhibitors- Captopril, lisinopril, enalapril, ramipril, benazepril Captopril (trade name capoten) - It is an oral drug belongs to ACE inhibitors.

Mechanism of Action-

ACE inhibitors are enzymes that inhibit the formation of angiotensin II, a potent vasoconstrictor. ACE, a membrane-bound dipeptidase dependent on zinc, facilitates the conversion of angiotensin I, a decapeptide, into angiotensin II, an octa-peptide with strong vasoconstrictive properties, by removing the C-terminal amino acids. ACE is a well-known enzyme that plays a crucial role in regulating blood pressure through the renin-angiotensin-aldosterone pathway.

Angiotensin II impacts blood pressure in several ways:

a. It stimulates the adrenal cortex, leading to increased aldosterone release. Aldosterone, in the kidney, enhances the reabsorption of sodium and water, subsequently increasing blood volume and blood pressure.

b. Angiotensin II also stimulates the posterior pituitary gland, increasing the secretion of antidiuretic hormone (ADH). ADH, similarly in the kidney, promotes the reabsorption of sodium and water, further increasing blood volume and blood pressure.

c. Angiotensin II directly acts on Angiotensin II receptors found in vascular smooth muscles, causing vasoconstriction and elevating blood pressure.

ACE inhibitors function by inhibiting ACE itself, reducing the formation of angiotensin II and, consequently, lowering blood pressure.

Pharmacokinetics (ADME):

ACE inhibitors are typically administered orally before meals, with an absorption rate of approximately 60 to 75%. If taken after food, absorption decreases by 25 to 40%. About 25 to 30% of the drug binds to plasma proteins, primarily albumin. Metabolism primarily occurs in the liver, leading to the formation of metabolites like captopril-cystein disulfide and the disulfide dimer of captopril, which are subsequently eliminated through urine.

Adverse Drug Reactions (ADRs):

Common side effects of ACE inhibitors include skin rash, dry cough (resulting from the accumulation of bradykinins), hypotension, alterations in taste, constipation or diarrhea. These medications are not recommended during pregnancy or while breastfeeding due to the drug's ability to cross the placental barrier and enter breast milk.

Therapeutic Uses:

ACE inhibitors are prescribed for the treatment of high blood pressure and heart failure. They are also employed to prevent kidney damage associated with high blood pressure and diabetes mellitus..

Marketed preparations-

- Captopril 25mg tab

- Lisinopril 20mg tab,
- Enalapril 20mg tab,
- Ramipril 10 mg tab.
- Benazepril 10mg tab.

Pharmacology of Angiotensin Receptor Antagonists (ARBs) - Saralasin, Losartan, Telmisartan, Valsartan, Candesartan:

ARBs are a class of medications that inhibit the action of angiotensin II by blocking its binding to angiotensin II receptors on the muscle cells surrounding blood vessels. This results in the dilation of blood vessels and a reduction in blood pressure. One notable advantage of ARBs is that they do not cause the adverse effect of dry cough, which is associated with ACE inhibitors.

Losartan:

Mechanism - Angiotensin II receptors, known as A1 receptors, are present in various tissues, including the heart, blood vessels, kidney, adrenal cortex, lung, and brain. Angiotensin II is the ligand that binds to these receptors. A1 receptors are part of the G protein-coupled receptor family (Gq). When Angiotensin II binds to A1 receptors, it activates phospholipase C (PLC), leading to an increase in intracellular calcium through second messengers like IP3 and DAG. The elevated calcium binds to the Calmodulin complex, which stimulates myosin light chain kinase (MLCK). This, in turn, leads to the phosphorylation of myosin light chains (MLC-P), resulting in vasoconstriction and increased blood pressure. Losartan, an ARB, works by blocking these A1 receptors, causing vasodilation and a decrease in blood pressure.

Pharmacokinetics (ADME) - Losartan is well-absorbed and undergoes first-pass metabolism. Its systemic bioavailability is approximately 33%. In the bloodstream, it binds to plasma proteins, mainly albumin. Losartan is metabolized in the liver by Cytochrome P-450 enzymes, leading to the formation of a carboxylic derivative. Both the free drug and its metabolites are eliminated through urine.

Adverse Drug Reactions (ADRs) - Common ADRs include hypotension and tachycardia. Losartan can also stimulate vagal (parasympathetic nerve) activity, leading to bradycardia. Importantly, Losartan does not cause dry cough because it does not lead to the accumulation of bradykinin.

Therapeutic Uses - Losartan is primarily used to treat hypertension. It is also employed to prevent stroke in patients with heart disease and to prevent kidney disease in hypertensive patients with diabetes mellitus.

Market Preparations - Losartan is available in 100mg tablets. Other ARBs, such as Telmisartan and Candesartan, are also available in different strengths for various medical indications.

d. Angina pectoris and anti-anginal drugs classification

The mentioned drugs are used in the treatment of angina pectoris, a condition characterized by severe chest pain resulting from inadequate blood supply (and therefore oxygen supply) to the heart muscle, often caused by the blockage or spasm of coronary arteries. The primary cause of angina is coronary artery disease, which is typically the result of atherosclerosis affecting the cardiac arteries. Common risk factors for angina include smoking, diabetes, high cholesterol, hypertension, a sedentary lifestyle, and a family history of early-onset heart disease. These medications aim to alleviate the symptoms and manage the underlying causes of angina.

Types of angina pectoris- There are three types

1. **Stable angina**: In this type the atherosclerotic plaque and inappropriate vasoconstriction (caused by endothelial damage) reduce the blood vessel lumen diameter. Hence there is reduction of blood flow.

2. **Unstable angina**: In unstable angina, rapture of the plaque triggers platelet aggregation, thrombus formation, and vasoconstriction. Depending upon plaque rapture this leads to non-Q wave (non-ST elevation) or Q wave (ST elevation) MI.

3. **Varient angina**: In this type atherosclerotic plaques are absent, and ischemia is caused by intense vasospasm. It occurs more in younger women. Drugs used in angina pectoris:

1.**Organic nitrates**: Amyl nitrite, isosorbide dinitrate, isosorbide trinitrate (nitro glycerine), isosorbide mononitrate, erythrytol tetranitrate, pentaerythrytol tetranitrate.

2. **Beta blockers** (propranolol, atenolol, metoprolol), CCBs (verapamil, nifedipine, deltiazem), K+ channel openers(nicorandil). 3.Antiplatelet drugs: Dipyridamole, aspirin, pentoxyphyllin. Pharmacology of anti -anginal drugs.

1. **Organic nitrates**: Amyl nitrite, isosorbide dinitrate, isosorbide trinitrate (nitro glycerine), isosorbide mononitrate, erythrytol tetranitrate, pentaerythrytol tetranitrate.

2. **Beta blockers** (propranolol, atenolol, metoprolol), CCBs (verapamil, nifedipine, deltiazem), K+ channel openers(nicorandil).

3. **Antiplatelet drugs**: Dipyridamole, aspirin, pentoxyphyllin.

1.Organic nitrates:

MOA (Mechanism of Action):

Within the body, organic nitrates are chemically reduced to release NO. No is an endogenous signalling molecule that causes vascular smooth muscle relaxation. The various organic nitrates give rise to NO by different chemical and biochemical mechanisms. Organic nitrates have the chemical structure RNO2. The nitro group is reduced to form NO in the presence of specific enzymes and extracellular and intracellular reductants (e.g. thiols). The NO diffuses into the vascular smooth muscles. In the vascular smooth muscle cells the NO activates guanylyl cyclise (GC). The activated guanylyl cyclase increases the formation of cGMP (second messenger) from GTP. The cGMP activates myosin-LC phosphatase. The activated myosin-LC phosphatase causes the dephosphorylation of myosin-LC-(P) to myosin-LC. This relaxes the smooth muscle of coronary blood vessels and causes coronary vasodilatation.

9 Pharmacological actions of organic nitrates (nitro glycerine)

1. Vasodilatation: Organic nitrates dilate both arteries and veins. a. Venodilatation (dilatation of veins): This decreases venous return. This reduces preload and end diastolic volume and pressure (EDVP). This also decreases the cardiac output. This decreases the size of the ventricles, intraventricular pressure and reduction in ventricular wall tension. This decreases the oxygen demand.

b. Coronary circulation: The larger coronary arteries get dilated. Smaller coronaries in ischemic region are already dilated in response to ischemia (lactic acid, adenosine, PGI2). This increases the blood flow to ischemic areas.

c. Arterial dilatation: Dilatation of larger arteries lead to flushing, headache. Dilatation of small arteries-> decreases PR-> decreases the DBP-> postural hypotension, reflex tachycardia.

d. Net effect on circulation: Decrease in venous return, reduction in CO, decreased SBP and SBP. Postural hypotension, palpitation, reflex tachycardia, flushing, headache are the side effects of these actions.

2. Oxygen demand: It is decreased.

3. Other smooth muscles: Relaxation of smooth muscles of gall bladder, biliary, sphincter of oddi, bronchial, GIT, urinary tract.

4. Antiplatelet effect: Nitrates have some antiplatelet action also. ADME: Nitroglycerine (NTG) administered by sublingual route, oral, transdermal ointment, intravenous route. Amyl nitrite is given by inhalation route. Nitrates undergo rapid first pass metabolism. Sub lingual route: Quick onset of action, liver is bypassed; action is terminated by spitting out the tablet. This route is preferred for treating acute attack of angina pectoris. Oral route: Onset of action is about 90 min, duration- 3-6h. This route is used for long-term prophylaxis. IV- NTG- it is used in unstable angina, MI with LVF and in hypertensive emergencies. Instructions to the patient: Nitrates should be taken in sitting or supine position to avoid postural hypotension. The tablet should be spitted or swallowed once the pain subsides or headache occurs.

The use of vasodilator medications, like K+ channel openers such as Nicorandil, can lead to various adverse drug reactions **(ADRs).** Here are some of the potential ADRs associated with these drugs:

Due to Vasodilation (VD):

- Headache
- Giddiness
- Postural hypotension (a drop in blood pressure upon standing)
- Flushing (a warm, red skin sensation)
- Dizziness (including cloudiness of consciousness)

Tolerance:

Tolerance can develop with continuous use, which means the medication's effectiveness may decrease over time, necessitating higher doses for the same effect.

Dependence:

Sudden withdrawal of these vasodilator medications can have serious consequences, including vasospasm (constriction of blood vessels), the potential for myocardial infarction (heart attack), and even death. This highlights the importance of a gradual and supervised discontinuation of these drugs.

It's essential for individuals taking these medications to be aware of these potential ADRs and to follow their healthcare provider's guidance closely, especially when it comes to dosage adjustments and discontinuation to minimize risks.

Nicorandil, a vasodilator and K+ channel opener, has several medical uses due to its ability to relax blood vessels and improve blood flow. Here are some of its common uses:

1. **Angina Pectoris:** Nicorandil is frequently used to treat angina pectoris, a condition characterized by chest pain or discomfort caused by reduced blood flow to the heart muscles.

2. **Myocardial Infarction (MI):** It can be employed in the management of myocardial infarction, commonly known as a heart attack. This use aims to improve blood flow to the heart tissue.

3. **Left Ventricular Failure (LVF):** In cases of left ventricular failure, Nicorandil may be prescribed to help alleviate symptoms by reducing cardiac afterload and improving blood flow.

4. **Hypertensive Crisis:** Nicorandil can be used in hypertensive crises, where there is a sudden and severe elevation in blood pressure, to lower blood pressure and decrease the workload on the heart.

5. **Cyanide Poisoning:** In some situations, Nicorandil is used in the management of cyanide poisoning. It helps by dilating blood vessels, which may aid in improving oxygen delivery to tissues in cases of cyanide poisoning.

6. **Biliary Colic and Esophageal Spasm:** Nicorandil may also be used to treat conditions like biliary colic (gallbladder pain) and esophageal spasm, where its vasodilatory effects can help alleviate symptoms.

10 Beta blockers:

Beta blockers are often prescribed to manage stable angina. They work by decreasing heart rate (HR), reducing the force of contraction (FC), and lowering oxygen demand. However, it's essential to note that they do not dilate coronary arteries. In some cases, beta blockers can decrease the force of contraction to the point of incomplete systolic ejection, which can lead to an increase in end-diastolic volume/pressure (EDV/P), which can be a disadvantage. Sudden withdrawal of beta blockers can potentially precipitate a myocardial infarction (MI), so discontinuation should be done gradually.

It's generally preferred to use cardio-selective beta blockers, as they primarily target beta-1 receptors, which affect the heart, and are less likely to block beta-2 receptors that cause vasodilation. When both beta-1 and beta-2 receptors are blocked (as in non-selective blockers), it can lead to unopposed alpha-1 receptor activity, resulting in vasoconstriction. This can potentially precipitate variant (vasospastic) angina.

Beta blockers are useful in unstable angina and non-ST-elevation myocardial infarction (NSTEMI) as well.

Calcium channel blockers (CCBs), when used for stable (exertional) angina, help by reducing heart rate and cardiac force, decreasing the heart's oxygen demand. Different types of CCBs have various effects on blood vessels and the heart. For instance, verapamil and diltiazem are known to cause arterial dilation, leading to a reduction in afterload and oxygen demand. However, it's important to note that CCBs may also cause reflex tachycardia, which can be an adverse reaction.

Furthermore, CCBs promote coronary artery dilation, enhancing blood supply to the heart. This dilation occurs in both large and small coronary arteries, redistributing blood to both ischemic and non-ischemic areas of the heart. This increased blood supply is beneficial in alleviating angina symptoms..

2. Miscellaneous drugs:

K+ Channel Openers (e.g., Nicorandil):

K+ channel openers like Nicorandil are medications that serve as coronary dilators. They work by dilating both small and large coronary arteries. This dilation is achieved through hyperpolarization of vascular smooth muscles, which leads to relaxation. These drugs also exhibit nitrate-like actions to further aid in vasodilation. Some common adverse effects of K+ channel openers include headache, palpitations, dizziness, nausea, and vomiting. However, they are contraindicated in patients with left ventricular failure (LVF) and those with hypotension.

Antiplatelet Drugs (e.g., Aspirin):

Antiplatelet drugs, such as Aspirin, are essential in preventing platelet aggregation and, subsequently, thrombus formation. This action is crucial in reducing the development of atherosclerotic plaques in blood vessels. Aspirin works by inhibiting the cyclooxygenase (Cox I and II) enzymes, which decreases the formation of thromboxane A2 from arachidonic acid. Thromboxane A2, under normal circumstances, induces platelet aggregation by binding to its receptors on platelets.

Aspirin, particularly at low doses, is often prescribed after a heart attack (myocardial infarction or MI) to reduce the risk of recurrent attacks. It is also employed in both stable and unstable angina pectoris. Additionally, at lower doses, Aspirin is used long-term to prevent heart attacks, strokes, and blood clot formation. Its antiplatelet effects make it a crucial medication in cardiovascular health.

Anti-arrhythmic drugs;

Classification and mechanism of action,

Pharmacology of quinidine (A proto type sodium channel blocker).

d. **Antiarrythmic drugs**

Introduction

Arrhythmia means disturbance of rate, regularity, origin or conduction of cardiac impulse. Cardiac arrhythmia is a group of condition in which the heart rate is irregular, too fast or too slow. If the beat is more than 100beats/min then it is tachycardia, and if below 60 beats/min then it is bradycardia. There are four main types of arrhythmias- extra beats, supra-ventricular tachycardia, ventricular arrhythmia and brady-arrythmia.

a. Extra beats- There are two types- premature atrial contractions and premature ventricular contractions.

b. Supra ventricular tachycardia- It is due to improper electrical activity and is arises from sinuatrial node (SAN). The heart rate may increases to 200 beats / min. Supraventricular tachycardias include atrial fibrillation, atrial flutter and paroxysmal supraventricular tachycardia (PSVT). **c.**Ventricular arrhythmias- These include ventricular fibrillation and ventricular tachycardia.

d.Bradarrythmias- It is a type of arrhythmia in which the heart decreases below 60beats/min. 12 Electrical activity of heart Phase O: Rapid depolarization, resting potential is -90 mV. Opening of Na+ channel, Na+ gets accumulated, potential increases to +20mV. 13

Phase-1: Partial repolarization, due to stoppage of Na+ channel + transient outward K+. Voltage becomes 10 mV.

Phase-2: Plateau phase. Voltage remains + ve (inside) -> voltage gated Ca2+channels get open – influx of Ca2+ from ECF and sarcoplasmic reticulum. Closure of Ca2+ channels at the end.

Phase -3: Rapid repolarisation: is due to outward of K+ plus stoppage of Ca2+influx. Resetting of resting potential to -90mV.

Phase-4: Diastolic depolarization: It is due to slow inward of Na+ current. Electrical activity is disturbed in cardiac arrhythmias.

Classification of antiarrythmic drugs:

There are 5 classes of antiarrythmic drugs:

Class I. Membrane stabilizing agents. (Na+ channel blockage).

       a. Quinidine, procainamide,disopyramide,
       b. lidnocaine, tocainide, c.flecainide, encainide

Class II. β blockers: Propranolol, esmolol, sotalol Class III. K+ channel blockers: Amiodarone, bretylium

Class IV. CCBs: Verapamil, diltiazem

Class V. Others: Digitalis, atropine, isoprenaline, adenosine. Mechanisms of antiarrythmic drugs

Class I. Membrane stabilizing agents. (Na+ channel blockage). a.Quinidine, procainamide,disopyramide,

b.lidnocaine, tocainide,

c.flecainide, encainide It is a stereoisomer of quinine an alkaloid obtained from cinchona bark. It decreases the excitability of the cardiac muscle by blocking the sodium channels across the pace maker cells of the SAN and cardiac muscles. This decreases the rise of phase o in pacemaker cells. This also increases effective refractory period (ERP) and QT interval and prolongation of QRS, PR, and RR intervals. This also leads to prolonged repolarisation due to decreased K+ efflux. Thus heart rate decreases.

Class II. β blockers: Propranolol, esmolol, sotalol

MOA (Mechanism of Action):

They have two types of actions. Membrane stabilizing action (because of the blockage of Na+ channel, reduces inflow of Ca2+ ions during phase-0) and beta blocking action. They block the beta1 receptors present on the SAN and AVN. This decreases HR and force of heart 14 contraction. Due to blockage of β1 receptors, all the effects are antagonized. Thus HR, conduction velocity (CV) and automaticity (ability of the cardiac cells to depolarize spontaneously) is reduced, which in turn decreases the contractility of the myocardium. Class III. K+ channel blockers: Amiodarone, bretylium,sotalol Amiodarone: They act by blocking K+ channel. Because of this blockage the efflux of K+ ions from myocardial cells to interstitial fluid is restricted. This decreases the repolarisation. This increases the duration of each beat. In the ECG it increases the QT, PR and RR interval. Also block Na+, Ca2+ channel and blocks beta receptors. They decrease the conduction velocity.

Class IV.

CCBs: Verapamil, diltiazem Antiarrythmic action is due to voltage sensitive Ca2+ channels blockage. This decreases the conduction velocity of the cardiac impulse and decreases the heart rate. CCBs also cause VD of arteries and veins. There is reduction in PR and CO. They decreases both SBP and DBP,

ClassV. Others: Digitalis, atropine, isoprenaline, adenosine. Pharmacology of quinidine

Class I a**. Quinidine**- It is a stereoisomer of quinine an alkaloid obtained from cinchona bark. It decreases the excitability of the cardiac muscle by blocking the sodium channels across the pace maker cells of the SAN and cardiac muscles. This decreases the rise of phase o in pacemaker cells. This also increases effective refractory period (ERP) and QT interval and prolongation of QRS, PR, and RR intervals. This also leads to prolonged repolarisation due to decreased K+ efflux. Thus heart rate decreases. Other actions of quinidine- It has anti-malarial action, inhibition of skeletal muscle contractility. At higher doses it increases the contractions of uterus and GIT. ADME- Quinidine is almost completely absorbed from the GIT. However, because of hepatic first-pass effect, the bioavailability is about 70- 80%. But no difference observed between the rate of quinidine absorption, when given by intramuscular injection or oral absorption. About 70 to 80 % of the drug bound to plasma protein. Plasma protein is decreased in patients with chronic liver disease. Quinidine concentrations in liver are 10 to 30 times higher than those in plasma. 50 to 90% of quinidine is metabolized in the liver to hydroxylated products - eg.4-hydroxyquinidine. The principal metabolite is 3 hydroxyquinidine which exerts similar effects to quinidine. The metabolites and free drug eliminated through urine. **Preparations-** Quinidine gluconate 324mg controlled release (CR) tabs, quinidine sulfate 200mg, 300mg tabs.

ADRs(Adverse Drug Reaction)

1. Idiosyncratic reactions- fever, angioedema (swelling under the skin due to the vascular leakage), asthma, thrombocytopenia, hepatitis.

2. GIT- Nausea, vomiting and diarrhoea.

3. CVS- precipitates CCF

4. **Cinchonism**- ringing in ears, deafness, vertigo, headache, and visual disturbances. Drug interactions:

1. If it is given with digitalis, the quinidine displaced from its binding sites and increases the toxicity.

2. With vasodilators-> more vasodilation.

3. With diuretics-> hypokalemia.

4. With beta blockers/CCBs-> myocardial depression. S

Uses –

Used in supra-ventricular tachycardias- Atrial flutter, atrial fibrillation,

PSVT.

Drugs used for therapy of congestive cardiac failure (CCF); Classification and mechanism of action of drugs used for CCF, Pharmacology of digoxin.

15 c) Drugs used for therapy of Congestive Heart Failure Congestive Heart Failure: It is a chronic progressive condition that affects the pumping power of the heart muscles. Heart failure may be LVF, RVF or both. a. Left ventricular failure (LVF): when left ventricle fails to pump adequately, there is incomplete ejection of blood from the left ventricle. This results in decrease in cardiac output (CO). (Stroke volume x HR= CO 70x72= 5Lt). The decreased CO leads to the less blood supply to the body tissue. This causes fatigue and decreased tolerance to the exercise. The oxygenated blood remains in the left ventricle. This increase end systolic volume (more than 60ml). Ventricular filling continues and this leads to the dilatation of the ventricles. The length of the myocardial muscle fibers increases. This slowly develops into hypertrophy of myocardium (remodelling of heart) or enlargement of the ventricle. The dilated left ventricle fails to increase force of contraction. The accumulated blood within left ventricle leads to the development of back pressure. The blood goes back to the left atrium. The left atrial pressure increases. The oxygenated blood goes back to the lungs. This causes pulmonary congestion and pulmonary oedema. The fluid gets accumulated in the alveoli. This impairs the gas exchange and oxygenation of blood. This leads to hypoxia and breathlessness. The decreased supply of blood stimulates the sympathetic nerves. This increases HR, vasoconstriction and force of contraction (but this is not possible). The decreased CO decreases renal blood flow. This decreases urine output. This causes Na and water retention. This increases blood volume, increased load on the heart. This also stimulates the rennin-angiotension activity. The decreased CO also reduces cerebral blood flow. This causes confusion and coma. Right ventricular failure (RVF) - RVF occurs as a result of LVF. In RVF the deoxygenated goes back to the right atrium and into the superior and inferior venacava. The blood also goes to the liver through

hepatic vein. This leads to the congestion and enlargement of the liver (hepatomegally). The back flow also leads to peripheral oedema noticeable near the limbs. The RVF also leads to ascites (accumulation of the fluid in the abdomen leading to hanging abdomen)..

Drugs used in CCF:

1. **Cardiotonic drugs**: Cardiac glycosides- Cardiac glycosides are present in the digitalis plant. Eg. Digoxin, digitoxin, gitoxin, lanatoside, quabain. 16

2. **Vasodilators-**
   a. **ACE-I**: e.g. Captopril, enalapril and lisinopril.
   b. ARBs (Angiotensin receptor antagonist) e.g Losartan.
   c. **Nitrovasodilators (organic nitrates)**- e.g. Glyceryltrinitrate (isosorbide trinitrate), isosorbide dinitrate.
   d. **Direct vasodilators**: e.g.Sodium nitroprusside, Hydralazine and nicorandil.
   e. **CCBs**: e.g .Nifedipine, and Amlodipine.
   f. **Phosphodiesterase III inhibitors**: e.g.Amrinone, milrinone.

3. **Adrenergic receptor antagonists**- Prazosin (α1 blocker), phentolamine (α1and α2 blocker).

4. **β1 receptor agonists**- Dobutamine.

5. **Diuretics**- e.g. Hydrochlorthiazide, frusemide and amiloride.

Pharmacology of digoxin- Digoxin is the purified cardiac glycoside extracted from the plant digitalis lanata.

1. **Cardiotonic drugs**: Cardiac glycosides- Cardiac glycosides are present in the digitalis plant. Eg. Digoxin,digitoxin,gitoxin, lanatoside,quabain. Digitalis: Two sources of digitalis are D.purpura, D.lanata. The important glycosides present in digitalis are digitoxin, gitoxin, digoxin, lanatoside. They are steroidal glycosides containing steroid nucleus. Each glycoside is made up of an aglycone (genin) and a sugar. The aglycon part is responsible for its pharmacological activity. The sugar part increases the pharmacokinetic properties like water solubility, cell permeability and potency of the aglycone. Pharmacological actions of Digoxin:

1. **Heart**: a. Force of Contraction: It is increased. This is known as +ve ionotropic effect. Contractions are more powerful. The duration for the systole decreases and for the diastole it is increases. There is more complete emptying. This increases cardiac output (CO) and reduces the size of the chambers.

(i) *Better tissue perfusion*. The increased CO results in decreased sympathetic tone. It reduces the heart rate, vasoconstriction.

(ii) *Increase in renal flow*- The increased CO also increases urine output. This decreases circulating volume, decrease in edema.

(iii) *Better emptying of the left ventricle*- This reduces the back pressure, pulmonary pressure. This decreases pulmonary edema. This improves breathlessness problem. Increase in FC and CO by digitalis is without corresponding increase in oxygen demand.

b. Heart Rate (HR) is decreased due to increase in cardiac output (CO) and decrease in sympathetic tone. The decreased HR is also due to the stimulation of vagus (parasympathetic) nerve by the digitalis c. Electrophysiological effects: Reduces SAN automaticity (vagal action + direct action at toxic doses). In AV node it decreases CV (conduction velocity). In the ventricles it increases automaticity. Increase in excitability. On ECG digitalis prolongs PR interval and depresses the ST segment. 17

2. **Kidneys**: Increase in urine output- secondary to increase in CO (digitalis does not have diuretic action or direct action on kidneys).

3. **CNS**: Higher doses activate chemoreceptor trigger zone (CTZ present in the medulla oblongata and is communicated with vomiting centre to initiate vomiting) and causes nausea, vomiting. Other CNS actions due to higher doses of digitalis are hallucinations, visual disturbances, disorientation, mental confusion, etc. MOA: The cardiac glycosides (digoxin) act by inhibiting the Na^+-K^+ ATPase enzyme activity (pump). This enzyme present on the myocardial cells. This pump ensures the transmembrane stransfer of the cations Na^+ and K^+. This pump consists of two alpha catalytic subunits and of two beta subunits. This pump uses the energy released by the hydrolysis of the ATP in the presence of magnesium to ensure the transport of Na^+ ions to outside the cells and of K^+ ions to inside. The inhibited enzyme cannot exchange Na^+ ions for K^+ ions. Thus all Na^+ ions remain inside the cell and its

concentration is increased in the cardiac muscle. Increased concentration of Na+ increases the transportation of Ca2+ from extracellular fluid (ECF) into the cell across the cell membrane by Na+/Ca2+ exchange mechanism. One molecule of extracellular Ca2+ is exchanged for 3 molecules of intracellular Na+. Increased concentration of intracellular Ca2+ triggers the release of large amounts of Ca2+ from the internal stores of sarcoplasmic reticulum into cytoplasm. Thus more of Ca2+ is available inside the cell. The Ca2+ bind with the binding site present on the troponin, this disturbs the troponin-tropomycin system. This causes the interaction of actin-myosin contractile proteins and brings about myocardial contraction.

Advantage of digitalis is that it increases force of contraction without increasing corresponding increase in the O2 demand. ADME- About 70 to 80% of oral dose of digoxin is absorbed, mainly in the intestine. The degree of binding to serum albumin is 20 to 30%. Digoxin is extensively distributed in the tissues-heart, kidney and skeletal muscles. The main route of elimination is renal excretion. About 25 to 28% of digoxin is eliminated by non renal routes. Nearly all of the digoxin is eliminated unchanged, with a small part as active metabolites.

ADRs(Adverse Drug Reaction):

1. Anorexia, nausea, vomiting- due to gastric irritation + stimulation of CTZ.

2.CNS: Headache, malaise (uneasiness), fatigue, drowsiness, weakness, paresthesia (abnormal sensation), disorientation, confusion, delirium (acute confusional state), hallucinations, convulsions.

3. Cardiac adverse effects: sinus bradycardia (due to increase vagal tone), AV block (partial or complete).

Drug interactions:

1. With quinidine increases the blood levels of digoxin by decreasing tissue binding of digoxin.

2. With amphotericin B results in hypokalemia, this increases digoxin toxicity.

3. With calcium increase the toxicity of digoxin.

4. With antacid digoxin absorption decreases.

5. With pentobarbitone metabolism of digoxin increases and decreases its toxicity.

6. With srythromycin digoxin metabolism decreases and toxicity increases. CI: Hypokalemia, hypercalcemia

Uses:

1. Congestive cardiac failure

2. Left ventricular failure

3. Paroxysmal supraventricular failure (PSVT)

4. Atrial flutter

5. Atrial fibrillation. Preparations- Digoxin tabs, inj Drugs used in treatment of hyperlipidaemias; Hyperlipidemia- It is a disorder which occurs due to the elevated levels of lipids (cholesterol and triglycerides) in the blood.

There are two types- **hypercholesterolemia and hypertriglyceridemia**. Hypercholesterolemia- It is due to high cholesterol in the blood. *Hypertriglyceridemia*. It is due to high triglycerides in the blood. *Hypercholesterolemia-* Cholesterol is a sterol (steroid alcohol). Cholesterol is essential for the formation of cell membrane, vit D, steroid hormones and bile acids. Since cholesterol is insoluble in water, it is transported in the blood in the form of lipoproteins. Lipoproteins are classified on the basis of density into- *VLDL, LDL, IDL* and *HDL*. All lipoproteins carry cholesterol, but elevated levels of the lipoproteins other than HDL are associated with an increased risk of atherosclerosis and coronary heart disease. The higher levels of HDL cholesterol are protective. Long term elevated levels of cholesterol results in atherosclerosis. This may lead to stenosis (narrowing) and occlusion of the arteries. A sudden occlusion of a coronary artery results in a myocardial infarction or heart attack. An occlusion of an artery supplying brain can cause a stroke. Hypercholesterolemia also leads to **xanthelasma palpebrarum** (yellowish patches near the eyelids, xanthomas (deposition of yellowish cholesterol rich material). Normal total cholesterol is 180-200mg/dL. xanthoma 19 Hypertriglyceridemia- Elevated levels of triglycerides also associated with atherosclerosis even in absence of hypercholesterolemia. Very high triglyceride levels also increase the risk of acute pancreatitis, xanthomas.

DRUGS USED IN LIPID DISORDERS- ANTI-HYPERLIPIDEMIA -

Hyperlipidemia refers to elevated levels of lipids (fats) in the bloodstream. It is a significant risk factor for cardiovascular diseases, including atherosclerosis, coronary artery disease, and stroke. Hyperlipidemia can manifest as elevated levels of various types of lipids, including cholesterol and triglycerides. Here's an overview of hyperlipidemia:

Types of Lipids in the Blood:

Cholesterol: Cholesterol is a waxy, fat-like substance that is present in the cells of the body and is essential for various functions. However, elevated levels of low-density lipoprotein (LDL) cholesterol, often referred to as "bad" cholesterol, are associated with an increased risk of atherosclerosis and heart disease. High-density lipoprotein (HDL) cholesterol is considered "good" cholesterol because it helps remove LDL cholesterol from the bloodstream.

Triglycerides: Triglycerides are a type of fat found in the blood. High levels of triglycerides are also associated with an increased risk of cardiovascular disease.

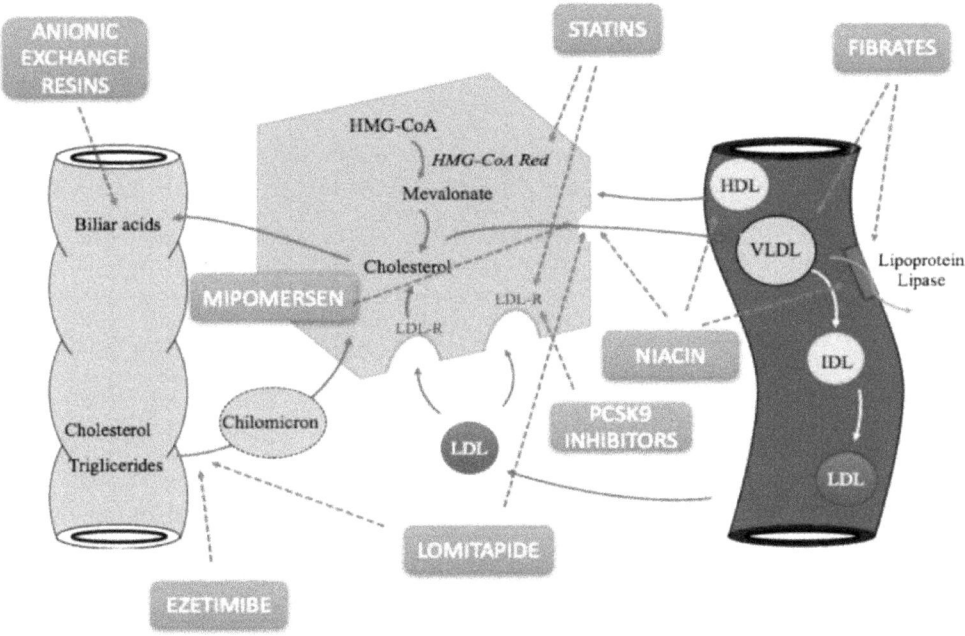

Fig.5 Drugs used in Lipid disorders

Classification:

Drug Class	Mechanism of Action	Examples
Statins (HMG-CoA Reductase Inhibitors)	Inhibit the enzyme HMG-CoA reductase, reducing cholesterol synthesis.	Atorvastatin, Simvastatin, Rosuvastatin
Bile Acid Sequestrants	Bind to bile acids in the intestine, preventing their reabsorption and increasing excretion.	Cholestyramine, Colesevelam, Colestipol
Fibrates	Activate peroxisome proliferator-activated receptor alpha (PPAR-alpha), reducing triglycerides and increasing HDL cholesterol.	Fenofibrate, Gemfibrozil
Niacin (Vitamin B3)	Mechanism not fully understood; increases HDL cholesterol and lowers LDL cholesterol.	Niacin (Nicotinic Acid)
Ezetimibe	Inhibits the absorption of cholesterol from the small intestine.	Ezetimibe

PCSK9 Inhibitors	Block the PCSK9 enzyme, increasing the number of LDL receptors on liver cells and reducing LDL cholesterol.	Evolocumab, Alirocumab
Omega-3 Fatty Acids	Reduce triglycerides and lower the risk of cardiovascular events.	Omega-3 supplements (e.g., fish oil)

1. **HMG-CoA reductase Inhibitors (Statins)**: pharmacological medicine of lipid-lowering medicine

Pharmacological actions and MOA:

During the synthesis of sterol, the 3-hydroxy 3- methyl radical glutaryl Co-enzyme A (HMG CoA) enzyme that converts HMG CoA to mevalonic acid. The mevalonic acid is then (after 20steps) regenerate into sterol. Statins act by inhibiting the HMG-CoA reductase, therefore sterol synthesis decreases. This ends up in increase expression of low-density lipoprotein receptors in hepatocytes. This will increase the uptake of IDL and low-density lipoprotein into the liver. Sterol biogenesis happens chiefly throughout sleep. Therefore statins ought to tend at bed time. Lipid-lowering medicine may be a long acting drug; this could tend at any time. Combination with cholestyramine or vitamin B complex enhances low-density lipoprotein lowering impact. Statins conjointly act by increasing the assembly of gas and this NO prevents the oxidisation of low-density lipoprotein. Grape fruits interferes the metabolism of statins and therefore the mixture ought to be avoided. ADME- Statins square measure administered orally. Most statins bind with plasma proteins. Most of administered statins endure initial pass impact. Solely 5-20% of the drug reaches the circulation. The statins square measure metabolized within the liver. The medication metabolites square measure excreted through the digestive juice and excretion.

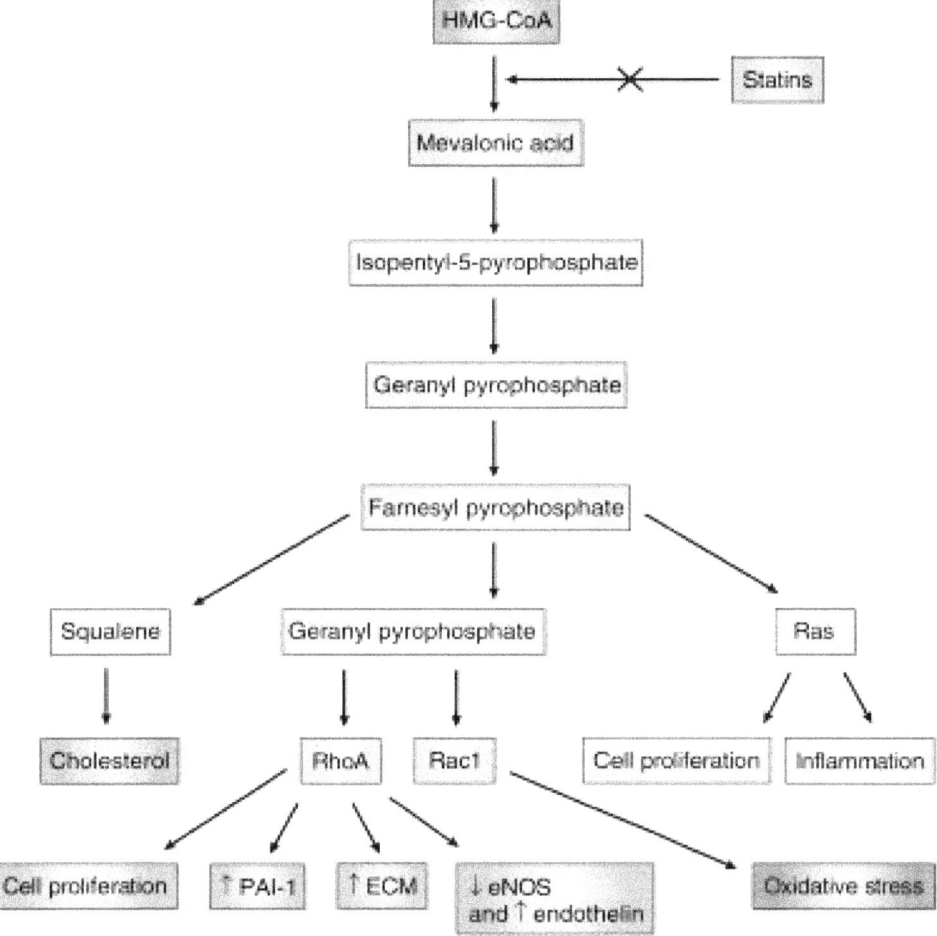

Fig.6 Mechanism of action HMG-CoA reductase Inhibitors (Statins)

ADRs (Adverse Drug Reaction):

1. Pathology syndrome- myodynia within the arms, legs and within the entire body.

2. Rhabdomyolysis- (Rapid breakdown of muscle tissue-release of myoglobin-> excretory organ toxicity thanks to its accumulation.)

3. Different common aspect effects: upset stomach (indigestion), flatulence (excessive gas within the GIT) and abdominal pain. Twenty

Therapeutic uses: Statins are a class of medications primarily used to manage and lower elevated levels of cholesterol in the blood. They are prescribed to reduce the risk of cardiovascular diseases, particularly in individuals with high cholesterol levels and those at risk of heart-related conditions. Some common therapeutic uses of statins include:

Lowering LDL Cholesterol: Statins are highly effective at reducing low-density lipoprotein (LDL) cholesterol, often referred to as "bad" cholesterol. By lowering LDL cholesterol levels, they help decrease the risk of atherosclerosis and coronary artery disease.

Reducing Cardiovascular Risk: Statins are prescribed to individuals with a high risk of heart attacks, strokes, and other cardiovascular events. They help lower the risk by decreasing the buildup of cholesterol plaques in the arteries.

Preventing Heart Attacks and Strokes: Statins are recommended for people who have already experienced a heart attack or stroke, as they can significantly reduce the risk of subsequent events.

Managing High Blood Pressure: Statins can help manage blood pressure by improving the health of the blood vessels and reducing inflammation.

Lowering Triglycerides: While their primary role is in reducing LDL cholesterol, statins can also have a modest effect on reducing triglyceride levels in the blood

Preventing Complications in Diabetes: Statins are used in individuals with diabetes to reduce the risk of complications, especially related to the heart and blood vessels.

Preventing Coronary Artery Disease: For those with a family history or genetic predisposition to coronary artery disease, statins can be used as a preventive measure

2. **Bile acid sequestrants** -: Cholestyramine, colestipol, Colesevalam

Medications interact with stomach acids and enhance the elimination of these acids through bowel movements. This, in turn, leads to increased excretion of fats in the stool. When the reabsorption of these stomach acids into the liver is inhibited, it triggers a rise in the conversion of cholesterol into stomach acids. This, in turn, stimulates cholesterol synthesis within the liver. As a result, more low-density lipoprotein receptors are expressed in the liver, leading to an increased uptake of low-density lipoprotein. Consequently, the level of low-density lipoprotein in the bloodstream decreases.

ADRs (Adverse Drug Reaction)

- Nausea, vomiting, constipation, bad taste, steatorrhea(presence of excess fat in feces), aggravation of hemorrhoids.
- Preparations and dose: Cholestyramine-12-24g/day, colestipol 15-30g/day. Uses - In hypercholesteremia.
- compound protein enzyme activators: medicine, medicinal drug, bezafibrate, finofibrate

MOA: The medication enhances the function of an extra-hepatic enzyme called lipoprotein lipase (LL), resulting in an increased breakdown of triglycerides from chylomicrons. This, in turn, lowers the levels of triglycerides in the bloodstream.

Regarding its pharmacokinetics (ADME), all fibrates are administered orally, and their absorption is more effective when taken with meals. Taking them on an empty stomach reduces absorption, with approximately 95% of the drug binding to plasma proteins, mainly albumin. Fibrates undergo metabolism in the liver, and the resulting metabolites are eliminated from the body through urine.

Therapeutic uses: Bile acid sequestrants are medications primarily used for the following therapeutic purposes:

Lowering Cholesterol: These drugs are employed to reduce elevated levels of cholesterol in the blood, especially low-density lipoprotein (LDL) cholesterol, often referred to as "bad" cholesterol.

Management of Hyperlipidemia: Bile acid sequestrants are prescribed to individuals with hyperlipidemia, a condition characterized by high levels of fats in the bloodstream. By lowering cholesterol levels, they help manage this condition and reduce the risk of cardiovascular diseases.

Coronary Artery Disease: They are used as part of the management plan for individuals with coronary artery disease (CAD) to lower the risk of heart-related events.

Adjunct to Lifestyle Modifications: Bile acid sequestrants are often recommended alongside lifestyle changes, such as adopting a heart-healthy diet and increasing physical activity.

Type 2 Diabetes Management: In some cases, these medications are used to help manage blood sugar levels in individuals with type 2 diabetes.

Lipoprotein-lipase activators (Fibrates):

Fibrates, which are derivatives of isobutyric acid, primarily stimulate the activity of an enzyme called lipoprotein lipase, a crucial protein involved in breaking down very low-density lipoprotein (VLDL), leading to a reduction in the current levels of triglycerides (TGs) in the bloodstream. This effect is achieved by activating peroxisome proliferator-activated receptor α (PPARα), a gene-regulating receptor expressed in the liver, adipose tissue, and muscles. Activation of PPARα enhances the synthesis of lipoprotein lipase and the oxidation of fatty acids. PPARα may also play a role in increasing the expression of low-density lipoprotein (LDL) receptors in the liver, particularly with second-generation fibrates like bezafibrate and fenofibrate. Additionally, fibrates reduce the synthesis of TGs in the liver, and they have a peripheral effect in reducing circulating free fatty acids.

Gemfibrozil, a derivative of fibric acid, is notably effective in reducing the levels of triglycerides (TGs) in the bloodstream by enhancing their breakdown and inhibiting their synthesis in the liver. In addition to its high efficacy in treating type III hyperlipidemia, gemfibrozil has also demonstrated positive effects in individuals with elevated blood cholesterol levels (hypercholesterolemia).

Pharmacokinetics:

- Gemfibrozil is totally absorbed orally, metabolized by glucuronidation and undergoes some enterohepatic circulation. it's excreted in urine; elimination t½ is 1–2 hour.

Adverse effects:

- Common aspect effects square measure epigastric distress, loose motions. Skin rashes, body ache, symptom, impotence, headache and blurred vision are reported.
- Myopathy is unusual.
- Gemfibrozil + medicine will increase risk of pathology. Incidence of bilestone isn't raised as was seen with medicine.
- It is contraindicated throughout gestation.

Lipolysis and triglyceride synthesis Inhibitor: Nicotinic acid

Mechanism of Action:

Lipid Modification: Nicotinic acid can effectively reduce levels of low-density lipoprotein (LDL) cholesterol, very low-density lipoprotein (VLDL) cholesterol, and triglycerides in the bloodstream while increasing high-density lipoprotein (HDL) cholesterol levels. This mechanism is not entirely understood but is thought to involve a decrease in the liver's production of VLDL cholesterol and an increase in the activity of lipoprotein lipase, which breaks down triglycerides.

Anti-Inflammatory Properties: Nicotinic acid has anti-inflammatory effects, which may contribute to its ability to lower cardiovascular risk. It can reduce the production of inflammatory substances in the body.

Therapeutic Uses:

Dyslipidemia Treatment: Nicotinic acid is primarily used for managing dyslipidemia, a condition characterized by abnormal levels of lipids (cholesterol and triglycerides) in the bloodstream. It is particularly effective in lowering LDL cholesterol and triglyceride levels while raising HDL cholesterol levels. Nicotinic acid is often prescribed to individuals with hypercholesterolemia and hypertriglyceridemia, as well as those with mixed hyperlipidemia.

Atherosclerosis and Cardiovascular Risk Reduction: Due to its lipid-modifying effects, nicotinic acid is employed to reduce the risk of atherosclerosis (narrowing and hardening of the arteries) and cardiovascular events, including heart attacks and strokes. It is often used in conjunction with lifestyle modifications, such as diet and exercise, to enhance its effectiveness.

Pellagra Prevention and Treatment: In the past, nicotinic acid was used to prevent and treat pellagra, a nutritional deficiency disease caused by a lack of niacin in the diet. However, it is now more commonly used for its lipid-modifying properties.

Adverse effects:

- The large doses needed for hypolipidaemic action are poorly tolerated. Only about half of the patients are able to take the full doses.

- Nicotinic acid is a cutaneous vasodilator: marked flushing, heat and itching (especially in the blush area) occur after every dose. This is associated with release of PGD2 in the skin, and can be minimized by starting with a low dose taken with meals and gradually increasing as tolerance develops.
- Dyspepsia is very common; vomiting and diarrhoea occur when full doses are given.
- Peptic ulcer may be activated.
- Dryness and hyperpigmentation of skin can be troublesome. Other long-term effects are: Liver dysfunction and jaundice.
- Serious liver damage is the most important risk. Hyperglycemia, precipitation of diabetes (should not be used in diabetics).
- It is contraindicated during pregnancy and in children.

Sterol absorption inhibitor:

Mechanism of Action:

Ezetimibe is a medication used to lower blood cholesterol levels and primarily acts through the following mechanisms:

Cholesterol Absorption Inhibition: Ezetimibe works by inhibiting the absorption of cholesterol from the small intestine. It specifically targets the Niemann-Pick C1-Like 1 (NPC1L1) protein, which is responsible for transporting cholesterol from the digestive tract into the bloodstream. By blocking this protein, ezetimibe reduces the absorption of both dietary cholesterol and cholesterol produced by the liver.

Decreased Cholesterol Delivery: By reducing the absorption of cholesterol, ezetimibe limits the amount of cholesterol delivered to the liver. This, in turn, triggers an increase in the expression of hepatic LDL receptors, leading to an increase in the clearance of low-density lipoprotein (LDL) cholesterol from the blood.

Therapeutic Uses:

Ezetimibe is prescribed for the following therapeutic purposes:

Hypercholesterolemia Management: Ezetimibe is primarily used to lower elevated levels of LDL cholesterol, often referred to as "bad" cholesterol. It is often prescribed as an adjunct to dietary and lifestyle modifications for individuals with hypercholesterolemia.

Familial Hypercholesterolemia: It is employed in the management of familial hypercholesterolemia, a genetic disorder characterized by extremely high cholesterol levels.

Mixed Hyperlipidemia: Ezetimibe may be used to treat individuals with mixed hyperlipidemia, a condition marked by elevated levels of both LDL cholesterol and triglycerides.

Prevention of Cardiovascular Events: Reducing LDL cholesterol with ezetimibe can help lower the risk of cardiovascular events, such as heart attacks and strokes.

Adverse Effects:

Common adverse effects associated with ezetimibe use may include:

Gastrointestinal Distress: This can include diarrhea, abdominal pain, and flatulence.

Fatigue: Some individuals may experience fatigue as a side effect.

Elevated Liver Enzymes: In rare cases, liver enzyme levels may increase. Regular monitoring of liver function is advisable.

Muscle Pain: Although muscle pain is less common with ezetimibe compared to statins, some individuals may still experience it.

DRUGS FOR NEURO-PSYCHIATRY DRUGS WORKING ON CNS

There are compounds of different chemical structures which cause hypnosis as physical sleeping.

Antidepressants:
- Fluoxetine (Prozac)
- Sertraline (Zoloft)
- Escitalopram (Lexapro)
- Venlafaxine (Effexor)

Antipsychotic Medications:
- Haloperidol (Haldol)
- Risperidone (Risperdal)
- Olanzapine (Zyprexa)
- Aripiprazole (Abilify)

Anxiolytics (Anti-Anxiety Medications):
- Diazepam (Valium)
- Lorazepam (Ativan)
- Alprazolam (Xanax)
- Clonazepam (Klonopin)

Mood Stabilizers:
- Lithium
- Valproic Acid (Depakote)

- Lamotrigine (Lamictal)
- Carbamazepine (Tegretol)

Antiepileptic Drugs (AEDs):

- Levetiracetam (Keppra)
- Topiramate (Topamax)
- Gabapentin (Neurontin)
- Pregabalin (Lyrica)

Stimulants:

- Methylphenidate (Ritalin)
- Amphetamine and Dextroamphetamine (Adderall)
- Lisdexamfetamine (Vyvanse)
- Sedatives and Hypnotics:
- Zolpidem (Ambien)
- Eszopiclone (Lunesta)
- Temazepam (Restoril)

Opioid Analgesics:

- Morphine
- Oxycodone (OxyContin)
- Hydrocodone (Vicodin)
- Fentanyl

Anticholinergics:

- Benztropine (Cogentin)
- Trihexyphenidyl (Artane)
- Nootropics and Cognitive Enhancers:
- Modafinil (Provigil)
- Piracetam (Nootropil)
- L-Theanine (commonly found in dietary supplements)

Barbiturates

Barbiturates are a class of drugs that act as central nervous system (CNS) depressants. They were widely used in the past for their sedative, hypnotic, and anticonvulsant properties. However, their use has decreased significantly over the years due to the development of safer and less addictive alternatives. Here are some key points about barbiturates:

Classification: Barbiturates are categorized based on how quickly they take effect and how long their effects last. Short-acting barbiturates, such as thiopental sodium, work within seconds and remain effective for approximately 30 minutes. They are primarily employed as intravenous aids during anesthesia.

On the other hand, long-acting barbiturates, like phenobarbital, have a duration of action lasting about 8 hours. These are valuable as sleep aids and sedatives, and when used in low doses, they can function as antiepileptic agents. However, they have a tendency to lead to a lingering drowsy feeling or "hangover." In contemporary clinical practice, phenobarbital is the primary barbiturate in use..

Mechanism of action: Barbiturates engage with barbiturate receptors located on a complex receptor-ion channel. Activation of GABA receptors leads to the opening of chloride channels, enabling chloride ions to enter the cell. This process hyperpolarizes the cell, resulting in reduced excitation. Barbiturates effectively decrease neuronal activity within the midbrain reticular formation, thus enhancing and prolonging the inhibitory effects of GABA and glycine. Additionally, they may inhibit the action of the excitatory neurotransmitter glutamic acid, and at high concentrations, sodium channels.

It's important to mention that barbiturates have a broader range of effects compared to benzodiazepines, which also display GABA-like actions. When the dosage of barbiturates is increased, it leads to a widespread depression of the central nervous system, as opposed to the specific depression observed at synaptic sites with benzodiazepines.

Pharmacokinetics: Within the domain of pharmacokinetics, which delves into the intricacies of drug movement within the body, barbiturates exhibit several distinctive attributes. These properties govern how these drugs are absorbed, distributed, metabolized, and ultimately eliminated from the body.

Firstly, when it comes to absorption, barbiturates are generally well-absorbed, particularly when administered orally. However, it's worth noting that the rate of absorption can differ among various types of barbiturates, with some being absorbed more quickly than others.

In terms of distribution, barbiturates exhibit a wide distribution throughout the body. They possess the ability to cross important barriers, such as the blood-brain barrier, which allows them to exert their effects within the central nervous system. Furthermore, these drugs can traverse the placental barrier, potentially affecting the developing fetus in pregnant individuals.

Metabolism is a crucial aspect of barbiturate pharmacokinetics. The liver plays a central role in metabolizing barbiturates, with involvement from various enzymes, including the cytochrome P450 system. It's important to note that the metabolites produced during this process are often less pharmacologically active than the parent compound.

Elimination of barbiturates primarily occurs through renal excretion, meaning that the drugs and their metabolites are expelled from the body via urine. The rate of elimination may vary among different barbiturates. Each barbiturate may have a distinct half-life, which determines the duration of its effects. Some barbiturates, known as short-acting, have relatively brief half-lives, while others, classified as long-acting, have a more prolonged duration of action.

A noteworthy feature of barbiturates is their potential to induce certain enzymes when used over an extended period. This enzyme induction typically occurs in the liver and can lead to increased metabolism of other drugs, potentially reducing their effectiveness.

Pharmacologic effects: Barbiturates are a class of drugs that act primarily on the central nervous system (CNS). Their effects can be divided into several key categories:

Sedation: Barbiturates are known for their sedative properties. They induce a calming and tranquilizing effect on the CNS, making them useful as sedative-hypnotic agents. They can help alleviate symptoms of anxiety, tension, and restlessness.

Hypnotic: At higher doses, barbiturates can induce sleep or a hypnotic state. They are used in medical practice as sleep aids for individuals with insomnia. However, their use for this purpose has significantly decreased due to safety concerns and the risk of dependence.

Anesthetic: Some barbiturates, especially the short-acting ones like thiopental, are used as intravenous anesthetics. They induce a rapid loss of consciousness and are employed during surgical procedures or in emergency situations.

Anticonvulsant: Barbiturates, such as phenobarbital, possess anticonvulsant properties. They can be prescribed to individuals with certain types of seizures or epilepsy to prevent or reduce the frequency of seizures.

Muscle Relaxation: Barbiturates can cause muscle relaxation, which can be beneficial for medical procedures that require muscle relaxation or for the management of muscle spasms.

Respiratory Depression: One of the most significant dangers associated with barbiturates is respiratory depression. In high doses or when combined with other depressant substances like alcohol, they can slow down breathing to a dangerous level, potentially leading to respiratory failure.

Hypotension: Barbiturates can lower blood pressure, which may be advantageous in certain medical situations but can also cause dizziness and fainting.

Adverse effects:

Cognitive Impairment: Barbiturates can impair cognitive function, including memory, attention, and problem-solving abilities. Prolonged use can lead to cognitive deficits.

Paradoxical Excitement: In some individuals, especially with high doses or when used recreationally, barbiturates can lead to paradoxical excitement, aggression, and impulsive behavior.

Drug Interactions: Barbiturates can interact with other medications, altering their effects. They may reduce the efficacy of certain drugs, such as oral contraceptives, and can interact with substances like alcohol.

GI Distress: Some individuals may experience gastrointestinal distress, including nausea, vomiting, and diarrhea, when taking barbiturates.

Liver and Kidney Damage: Long-term use of barbiturates can have adverse effects on the liver and kidneys, potentially leading to organ damage.

Skin Reactions: Allergic reactions and skin rashes are possible adverse effects of barbiturates.

Antiepileptic drugs

Sodium Channel Blockers: These drugs work by blocking sodium channels in neurons, reducing excessive electrical activity in the brain.

Examples: Phenytoin, Carbamazepine.

GABA Enhancers: These drugs enhance the effects of the inhibitory neurotransmitter GABA in the brain, reducing neuronal excitability.

Examples: Benzodiazepines (e.g., Diazepam), Barbiturates (e.g., Phenobarbital).

Calcium Channel Blockers: These drugs inhibit calcium channels and reduce the release of excitatory neurotransmitters.

Example: Ethosuximide.

Other Mechanisms: Some AEDs have unique mechanisms of action or affect different neurotransmitters to control seizures.

Example: Topiramate (Glutamate Inhibitor). There are anticonvulsant drugs of different actions:

I. Common action for cure acute convulsion of different etiology:

1. General anesthetic (phthorotanum, natrii oxybutyras);

2. Hypnotic drugs (chlorali hydras);

3. Tranquilizators (diazepamum);

4. Neuroleptics (aminazinum);

5. Magnesii sulfas;

6. Myorelaxants (as helping agents);

II. Specific drugs:

1. Drugs for treatment epilepsy;

2. Drugs for treatment Parkinson disease.

Mechanisms of Action: Mechanisms of Action of Antiepileptic Drugs (AEDs):

Voltage-Gated Sodium Channel Blockers: Some AEDs, like carbamazepine and phenytoin, work by blocking voltage-gated sodium channels. By doing so, they reduce the excessive and repetitive firing of action potentials in neurons.

Enhancement of GABAergic Inhibition: GABA (gamma-aminobutyric acid) is the primary inhibitory neurotransmitter in the brain. AEDs like benzodiazepines, phenobarbital, and natrii valproas enhance the inhibitory effects of GABA by interacting with GABA receptors or chloride ion channels. This leads to decreased neuronal excitability.

Inhibition of Glutamate Activity: Glutamate is the primary excitatory neurotransmitter in the brain. Some AEDs, like phenobarbitalum and topiramatum, act as antagonists at glutamate receptors, reducing excitatory signals in the brain.

Enhancement of GABA Levels: Vigabatrinum irreversibly inactivates GABA transaminase, an enzyme that breaks down GABA. By inhibiting this enzyme, it increases GABA levels, further enhancing inhibitory effects.

Inhibition of GABA Reuptake: Tiagabinum inhibits the reuptake of GABA by neurons and glia, increasing the availability of GABA in the synaptic cleft.

Low-Threshold (T-Type) Calcium Channel Blockers: Drugs like ethosuximide and natrii valproas inhibit low-threshold calcium channels, particularly in thalamic neurons. This action can help control seizures, especially absence seizures.

Potentiation of Potassium Channels: Natrii valproas can enhance potassium channel permeability, leading to neuronal membrane hyperpolarization and reduced excitability.

Structural Analogue of GABA: Gabapentin is a structural analogue of GABA, although it doesn't directly activate GABA receptors. Its exact mechanism of action is not fully understood, but it is thought to modulate calcium channels and influence excitatory neurotransmission.

Therapeutic uses: Epilepsy Management: Antiepileptic drugs are primarily used for the treatment of epilepsy. They help prevent or control seizures in individuals with epilepsy, allowing them to lead a more normal life. The choice of AED depends on the type of epilepsy and the patient's response.

Status Epilepticus: In cases of prolonged seizures or status epilepticus, where seizures last for an extended period, intravenous administration of AEDs like diazepam, lorazepam, or phenytoin can help terminate the seizure activity.

Neuropathic Pain: Some antiepileptic drugs, such as gabapentin and pregabalin, are used to manage neuropathic pain conditions. They can alleviate pain associated with diabetic neuropathy, post-herpetic neuralgia, and other chronic pain syndromes.

Bipolar Disorder: Certain AEDs, including valproic acid, lamotrigine, and carbamazepine, are used as mood stabilizers in the treatment of bipolar disorder. They help manage manic and depressive episodes.

Migraine Prophylaxis: AEDs like topiramate are used for the prevention of migraine headaches in individuals with frequent or severe migraines.

Trigeminal Neuralgia: Carbamazepine is often prescribed to relieve the severe facial pain associated with trigeminal neuralgia.

Alcohol Withdrawal: AEDs such as diazepam and chlordiazepoxide are used in alcohol withdrawal treatment to prevent seizures and manage withdrawal symptoms.

Anxiety Disorders: Clonazepam, a benzodiazepine AED, is sometimes used to manage anxiety disorders, particularly panic disorder and social anxiety disorder.

ADHD (Attention Deficit Hyperactivity Disorder): Some AEDs, like valproic acid, may be considered in the management of ADHD, especially in cases where other treatments are ineffective.

Neuromuscular Disorders: AEDs like phenytoin and carbamazepine can be used in the management of certain neuromuscular disorders, such as myotonia and neuromyotonia..

Phenytoin

Pharmacokinetics: Phenytoin works by stabilizing cell membranes through the reduction of sodium ion (Na+) conductance when neurons are firing excessively at high frequencies. Its suppressive effect specifically targets abnormal neuronal hyperactivity, allowing normal action potential conduction while stopping seizure activity. Phenytoin, classified as a weak acid, is subject to variable, incomplete, and sluggish absorption in the intestines. Approximately 90% of it binds to plasma proteins. The drug undergoes metabolism within the microsomal system and is eliminated first through the bile and subsequently through the urine.

Therapeutic uses: Phenytoin is employed for the following therapeutic purposes:

Management of seizures and epilepsy: Phenytoin is primarily utilized to prevent and control various types of seizures, including complex partial seizures, tonic-clonic seizures, and seizures occurring during neurosurgery.

Prevention of seizures in head injuries: It may be administered to prevent seizures that can occur following head injuries or brain trauma.

Cardiac arrhythmias: In some cases, phenytoin can be used to manage certain types of irregular heart rhythms, such as ventricular arrhythmias.

Adverse effects: The use of phenytoin may lead to various adverse effects. These can include:

Central Nervous System Effects: Phenytoin may cause dizziness, drowsiness, headache, and difficulty concentrating. In some cases, it can result in confusion, slurred speech, or mood changes.

Gingival Hyperplasia: Long-term use of phenytoin may lead to the overgrowth of gum tissue, known as gingival hyperplasia.

Diplopia: Some individuals may experience double vision or other visual disturbances.

Nystagmus: Phenytoin can cause rapid, involuntary eye movements.

Ataxia: It may lead to unsteady gait and coordination difficulties.

Hirsutism: Excessive hair growth in specific areas may occur.

Coagulation Issues: Phenytoin can affect blood clotting, increasing the risk of bleeding or bruising.

Hepatic Effects: Rarely, it may lead to liver problems, including elevated liver enzymes and hepatitis.

Dermatological Reactions: Skin reactions like rash, itching, and, in severe cases, a potentially life-threatening condition known as Stevens-Johnson syndrome may occur.

Osteomalacia: Long-term use can result in softening of the bones.

Teratogenicity: Phenytoin poses a risk of birth defects if used during pregnancy.

Interaction with Other Drugs: Phenytoin may interact with other medications and impact their effectiveness or safety.

Succinimides: Ethosuximide

Ethosuximide is an antiepileptic drug primarily used in the management of absence seizures. Here is some information on its mechanism of action, pharmacokinetics, and therapeutic uses:

Mechanism of Action:

Ethosuximide's precise mechanism of action is not entirely understood, but it is believed to affect calcium channels in thalamic neurons. These neurons are known for their role in generating rhythmic cortical discharges associated with absence seizures. Ethosuximide appears to reduce low-threshold (T-type) calcium currents in thalamic neurons, preventing the abnormal rhythmic firing of neurons seen in absence seizures.

Pharmacokinetics:

Absorption: Ethosuximide is well-absorbed after oral administration.

Distribution: It has a relatively short half-life and is distributed to various tissues in the body.

Metabolism: Ethosuximide undergoes hepatic metabolism.

Elimination: The drug and its metabolites are primarily excreted in the urine.

Therapeutic Uses:

The primary therapeutic use of ethosuximide is in the treatment of absence seizures, also known as petit mal seizures. It is considered the first-line treatment for this type of seizure. Ethosuximide helps control and reduce the frequency of absence seizures without significant sedative effects, making it particularly useful for pediatric patients.

It's important to note that ethosuximide is not effective in managing other types of seizures, and its use is generally limited to absence seizures due to its specific mechanism of action.

Benzodiazepines are a class of drugs with various medical uses, primarily for their anxiolytic (anxiety-reducing), sedative, muscle relaxant, and anticonvulsant properties. Mechanism of Action:

Benzodiazepines exert their effects by enhancing the actions of gamma-aminobutyric acid (GABA), which is an inhibitory neurotransmitter in the central nervous system. The key aspects of their mechanism of action include:

GABA Facilitation: Benzodiazepines bind to specific receptors on the GABAA receptor-chloride ion channel complex, which leads to an increase in the frequency of chloride ion channel opening. This enhances the inhibitory effects of GABA, effectively reducing neuronal excitability.

Duration of Chloride Ion Channel Opening: Benzodiazepines can enhance the duration of chloride ion channel opening by interacting with a particular receptor site. This further enhances the inhibitory actions of GABA.

CNS Depression: Increasing the dose of benzodiazepines results in a generalized depression of the central nervous system (CNS), affecting various synaptic sites, which contributes to their sedative effects.

Pharmacokinetics:

Absorption: Benzodiazepines are generally well-absorbed after oral administration, with varying rates of absorption depending on the specific drug.

Distribution: They distribute throughout the body, including the brain and other tissues.

Metabolism: Many benzodiazepines undergo hepatic metabolism, primarily by cytochrome P450 enzymes.

Elimination: They are primarily excreted in the urine as metabolites.

Adverse Effects:

Benzodiazepines are generally well-tolerated when used as prescribed. However, they can have side effects, especially when misused or taken in excess. Common adverse effects include:

Sedation: Many benzodiazepines can cause drowsiness or sedation, which can affect a person's ability to drive or operate heavy machinery.

Tolerance and Dependence: Prolonged use of benzodiazepines can lead to tolerance, meaning higher doses are needed to achieve the same effect. This can also result in physical and psychological dependence.

Cognitive Impairment: These drugs can impair cognitive function, affecting memory and concentration.

Withdrawal Symptoms: Abrupt discontinuation after prolonged use can lead to withdrawal symptoms, which may include anxiety, insomnia, tremors, and seizures in severe cases.

Potential for Misuse: Benzodiazepines have a potential for misuse and addiction when used outside of medical supervision.

Therapeutic use:

Anxiety Disorders: Benzodiazepines are used to alleviate symptoms of generalized anxiety disorder (GAD), panic disorder, and social anxiety disorder. They provide rapid relief from acute anxiety but are generally prescribed for short-term use due to the risk of dependence.

Insomnia: Benzodiazepines can be used as short-term sleep aids for individuals with insomnia. They help induce sleep and improve sleep maintenance.

Seizures: Some benzodiazepines, such as diazepam and lorazepam, are used to manage seizures, especially in emergency situations. They have anticonvulsant properties.

Muscle Relaxation: Benzodiazepines like diazepam and lorazepam are prescribed for muscle spasms, tension, and related conditions. They relax skeletal muscles and reduce muscle spasticity.

Sedation and Premedication: Benzodiazepines may be used before medical procedures or surgery to induce sedation and reduce anxiety in patients. They can also be used for sedation in intensive care units.

Alcohol Withdrawal: Benzodiazepines are sometimes used to manage symptoms of alcohol withdrawal, such as seizures and agitation.

Status Epilepticus: In emergency situations where individuals experience prolonged seizures (status epilepticus), benzodiazepines like diazepam are administered intravenously to stop the seizures.

Agitation and Aggression: They can be used to manage acute agitation and aggression in psychiatric or medical settings.

Relief from Delirium: In some cases, benzodiazepines may be used to alleviate symptoms of delirium, especially in patients with underlying conditions like dementia.

Adverse effects: Diplopia, ataxia, and nausea, bone marrow depression, including aplastic anemia, congestive heart failure, atropine-like symptoms, kidney and liver toxicity may occur.

Sodium valproate is a medication with several mechanisms of action and is used to treat various medical conditions.

Mechanism of Action:

Gamma-Aminobutyric Acid (GABA) Enhancement: Sodium valproate enhances the action of GABA, a neurotransmitter that has inhibitory effects on the central nervous system. By increasing GABA levels, it helps reduce excessive neuronal excitation and prevent seizures.

Voltage-Gated Sodium Channels: Sodium valproate also has sodium channel-blocking properties. It can limit the repetitive firing of neurons by blocking voltage-gated sodium channels, which play a role in generating action potentials. This effect contributes to its antiepileptic action.

Pharmacokinetics:

Absorption: Sodium valproate is well-absorbed after oral administration.

Distribution: It has a wide distribution in the body, including the central nervous system.

Metabolism: It undergoes hepatic metabolism and is metabolized to its active form, valproic acid.

Elimination: The drug is excreted primarily through the urine.

Therapeutic Uses:

Epilepsy: Sodium valproate is primarily used in the treatment of various types of epileptic seizures, including absence seizures, complex partial seizures, and generalized tonic-clonic seizures. It is effective in both adults and children.

Bipolar Disorder: Sodium valproate is also prescribed to manage bipolar disorder, helping to stabilize mood and prevent mood swings in individuals with this condition.

Migraine Prophylaxis: It can be used to prevent recurring migraine headaches.

Mania: In some cases, sodium valproate is used to manage manic episodes in bipolar disorder.

Adverse Effects:

Gastrointestinal Distress: Common side effects include nausea, vomiting, and abdominal pain.

Sedation: It may cause drowsiness or sedation.

Weight Gain: Some individuals may experience weight gain.

Tremor: Hand tremors are possible, especially at high doses.

Liver Effects: Sodium valproate can affect liver function, and regular monitoring of liver enzymes may be necessary during treatment.

Thrombocytopenia: It may cause a reduction in blood platelets.

Pancreatitis: Rarely, it can lead to pancreatitis, characterized by severe abdominal pain.

The newer generation

Vigabatrin (VGB)

Vigabatrin (VGB) is an antiepileptic drug with distinct mechanisms of action and is used to manage certain types of seizures.

Mechanism of Action:

Vigabatrin primarily exerts its antiepileptic effects through a unique mechanism:

GABA Transaminase Inhibition: Vigabatrin irreversibly inhibits the enzyme GABA transaminase. This enzyme is responsible for the breakdown of the inhibitory neurotransmitter gamma-aminobutyric acid (GABA). By inhibiting GABA transaminase, vigabatrin increases GABA levels in the brain, enhancing its inhibitory effects on neuronal activity. This helps reduce the likelihood of seizures, particularly in conditions where excessive neuronal excitation is a problem.

Felbamate (FBM) is an antiepileptic drug with distinct mechanisms of action and therapeutic uses. Here are the key details about felbamate:

Mechanism of Action:

Felbamate's mechanism of action is not fully understood but is believed to involve several modes of action, including:

Blockade of NMDA Receptors: Felbamate is known to antagonize N-methyl-D-aspartate (NMDA) receptors, which play a role in excitatory neurotransmission in the brain. By blocking these receptors, it reduces excessive neuronal excitation.

Enhancement of GABAergic Inhibition: Felbamate may enhance the inhibitory effects of gamma-aminobutyric acid (GABA), the primary inhibitory neurotransmitter in the brain, by increasing its binding to GABA receptors.

Blockade of Sodium Channels: It may also exert some of its effects by blocking voltage-gated sodium channels in neuronal membranes, which reduces neuronal excitability.

Agents used in the treatment of Parkinsonian disorders

The classification of these drugs includes:

Dopaminergic Medications:

Levodopa (L-DOPA): Levodopa is a precursor of dopamine and is the most effective medication for managing Parkinson's disease symptoms. It is often combined with other drugs to enhance its effectiveness.

Dopamine Agonists: These drugs stimulate dopamine receptors directly, and they can be used as monotherapy or in combination with levodopa.

Examples: Pramipexole, Ropinirole, Rotigotine.

Enzyme Inhibitors:

Carbidopa: Administered in combination with levodopa (Sinemet) to prevent the peripheral breakdown of levodopa before it reaches the brain.

Entacapone: Used with levodopa to extend its duration of action by inhibiting the peripheral metabolism of levodopa.

Anticholinergic Medications:

These drugs help reduce the symptoms of tremors and muscle rigidity in Parkinson's disease by blocking the effects of acetylcholine, which is in excess in the brains of people with Parkinson's.

Examples: Benztropine, Trihexyphenidyl.

Monoamine Oxidase B (MAO-B) Inhibitors:

MAO-B inhibitors block the enzyme MAO-B, which breaks down dopamine in the brain. By inhibiting MAO-B, these drugs help maintain dopamine levels.

Examples: Selegiline, Rasagiline.

Catechol-O-Methyltransferase (COMT) Inhibitors:

COMT inhibitors help prolong the effects of levodopa by inhibiting the breakdown of levodopa in the body.

Examples: Tolcapone, Entacapone.

Antiviral Agents:

Some antiviral agents, such as amantadine, are used to manage symptoms of Parkinson's disease.

Adenosine A2A Receptor Antagonists:

These drugs are relatively new additions to the treatment of Parkinson's disease, and they work by blocking specific receptors in the brain.

Examples: Istradefylline.

Surgical Treatments:

Surgical procedures, such as deep brain stimulation (DBS), are sometimes used to treat Parkinsonian disorders. Electrodes are implanted in specific brain areas, and electrical impulses are used to control symptoms.

Supportive and Symptomatic Treatments:

Various medications may be used to address specific symptoms or complications associated with Parkinson's disease, such as depression, anxiety, and sleep disturbances.

Mechanism of Action - Levodopa (L-DOPA): Levodopa is a precursor of dopamine, a neurotransmitter in the brain. It crosses the blood-brain barrier and is converted into dopamine in the brain. Dopamine deficiency is a key factor in Parkinson's disease. By increasing dopamine levels in the brain, levodopa helps improve motor function and reduce the symptoms of Parkinson's disease.

Pharmacokinetics - Levodopa (L-DOPA): Levodopa is well absorbed from the gastrointestinal tract and rapidly crosses the blood-brain barrier. It is metabolized in the periphery and central nervous system to form dopamine. Levodopa's effects can be influenced by dietary protein intake and the presence of other medications.

Therapeutic Effects - Levodopa (L-DOPA): Levodopa is the most effective drug for alleviating the motor symptoms of Parkinson's disease, including bradykinesia, rigidity, and tremors. It can significantly improve the quality of life for individuals with Parkinson's disease and enhance their ability to perform daily activities.

Adverse Effects - Levodopa (L-DOPA): While levodopa is highly effective, long-term use can lead to motor fluctuations, dyskinesias (involuntary movements), and wearing-off phenomena, where the medication's effects wear off before the next dose. Additionally, levodopa can cause nausea, vomiting, orthostatic hypotension, and psychiatric side effects.

Mechanism of Action - Carbidopa is often used in combination with levodopa in the treatment of Parkinson's disease. It does not have a direct therapeutic effect on its own. Instead, its primary role is to enhance the effectiveness of levodopa therapy. Carbidopa inhibits the enzyme aromatic L-amino acid decarboxylase (AADC) both in the peripheral tissues and the central nervous system, preventing the conversion of levodopa to dopamine outside of the brain. This inhibition ensures that more levodopa reaches the brain, where it can be converted to dopamine, which is deficient in Parkinson's disease.

Pharmacokinetics - Carbidopa is typically administered orally alongside levodopa. It is rapidly absorbed from the gastrointestinal tract and, like levodopa, can cross the blood-brain barrier. It has a relatively short half-life and is excreted primarily in the urine.

Therapeutic Effects Carbidopa enhances the therapeutic effects of levodopa by allowing more levodopa to reach the brain. As a result, it helps improve motor function and reduce the symptoms of Parkinson's disease, similar to levodopa.

Adverse Effects - Carbidopa itself does not produce significant adverse effects when used in combination with levodopa. The adverse effects experienced are often related to levodopa therapy, including motor fluctuations, dyskinesias, nausea, orthostatic hypotension, and psychiatric side effects. Carbidopa primarily serves to minimize these side effects by allowing lower doses of levodopa to be used for optimal therapeutic effect.

Anticholinergic agents decrease the excitatory actions of cholinergic neurons on cells in the striatum by blocking muscarinic receptors.

Pharmacologic effects: Drugs such as cyclodolum, troparinum, brinerdinum may improve the tremor and rigidity of Parkinsonism but they have little effect on bradykinesia. They are used adjunctively in Parkinsonism; they also alleviate reversible extrapyramidal symptoms caused by antipsychotic drugs.

Therapeutic uses: While not as effective as laevodopum or bromocriptinum, anticholinergic agents may have an additive therapeutic effect at any stage of the disease when taken concurrently.

Adverse effects such as mental confusion and hallucinations due to central muscarinic toxicity, can occur as can peripheral atropine-like toxicity (e.g. cycloplegia, urinary retention, and constipation).

Selegiline:

Mechanism of Action - Selegiline: Selegiline is an irreversible and selective inhibitor of monoamine oxidase B (MAO-B) enzyme. It prevents the breakdown of dopamine in the brain by inhibiting the MAO-B enzyme, which is responsible for metabolizing dopamine. By preserving dopamine levels, selegiline helps to maintain dopaminergic activity in the brain, which is often reduced in Parkinson's disease. This mechanism contributes to the alleviation of Parkinson's disease symptoms.

Pharmacokinetics - Selegiline: Selegiline can be administered orally and is well-absorbed from the gastrointestinal tract. It is metabolized in the liver to metabolites, including L-amphetamine and L-methamphetamine. These metabolites are excreted in the urine. The pharmacokinetics of selegiline can vary based on the formulation used, such as oral tablets or transdermal patches.

Therapeutic Effects - Selegiline: Selegiline is used as an adjunctive treatment in Parkinson's disease. By inhibiting MAO-B, it helps to maintain dopamine levels, thereby reducing the motor symptoms of the disease, such as tremors, rigidity, and bradykinesia. It is often used in combination with levodopa.

Adverse Effects -Common adverse effects of selegiline are mild and include gastrointestinal symptoms like nausea. However, when used in high doses or inappropriately, it can lead to side effects similar to amphetamines, such as restlessness, insomnia, and elevated blood pressure. It is important to follow the prescribed dosing regimen to minimize these adverse effects. The transdermal formulation can also minimize some side effects associated with the oral form.

Catechol-O-methyltransferase (COMT) inhibitors, such as

Entacapone, work by blocking the action of the COMT enzyme, which is responsible for breaking down certain neurotransmitters, including dopamine, in the brain. By inhibiting COMT, these drugs help maintain higher levels of dopamine, which is essential for controlling movement and other functions.

In terms of pharmacokinetics, COMT inhibitors are generally well-absorbed after oral administration. They are metabolized in the liver and excreted in the urine.

COMT inhibitors are used in conjunction with levodopa for the treatment of Parkinson's disease. By prolonging the action of levodopa, they help manage the motor symptoms of the disease more effectively.

Adverse effects of COMT inhibitors can include gastrointestinal disturbances, such as diarrhea and nausea. In some cases, they may lead to an increase in certain liver enzymes.

Antipsychotic agents

These agents are prescribed for the management of psychotic symptoms; they are sometimes referred to as **major tranquilizers** or **neuroleptics.** They are useful in both acute and chronic psychoses and in nonpsychotic individuals who are delusional or excited. They improve mood and behavior without producing excessive sedation. As a group, these agents produce little physical dependence or habituation but to greater extent they are capable of causing extrapyramidal symptoms, both reversible (Parkinsonian symptoms, akathisia) and irreversible (tardive dyskinesia). The antipsychotic drugs **(neuroleptics)** are effective in controlling many manifestations of psychotic illness. Hallucinations or delusions, may be attenuated by antipsychotic drugs.

Antipsychotic agents, also known as antipsychotic drugs or neuroleptics, are medications used to treat various psychiatric conditions, including schizophrenia, bipolar disorder, and other psychotic disorders. Here is a list of some antipsychotic agents:

Typical Antipsychotics (First-generation antipsychotics):

- Haloperidol
- Chlorpromazine

- Fluphenazine
- Perphenazine
- Trifluoperazine
- Thioridazine
- Loxapine
- Pimozide

Atypical Antipsychotics (Second-generation antipsychotics):

- Risperidone
- Olanzapine
- Quetiapine
- Aripiprazole
- Ziprasidone
- Clozapine
- Lurasidone
- Asenapine
- Paliperidone

Mechanism of Action:

Typical antipsychotics primarily block dopamine receptors in the brain. They are dopamine receptor antagonists, specifically targeting D2 receptors. By reducing the activity of dopamine, they help alleviate the positive symptoms of schizophrenia, such as hallucinations and delusions.

Pharmacokinetics:

The pharmacokinetics of typical antipsychotics can vary between individual drugs. They are generally well-absorbed after oral administration and reach peak plasma concentrations within a few hours. They are highly protein-bound in the bloodstream. Most are extensively metabolized in the liver, and their metabolites are often pharmacologically active. Excretion typically occurs through urine.

Therapeutic Uses:

Typical antipsychotics are primarily used for the treatment of psychotic disorders, including schizophrenia and bipolar disorder. They are effective in managing positive symptoms, such as hallucinations, delusions, and thought disorders. Some typical antipsychotics are also used to manage severe anxiety and agitation.

Adverse Effects:

Typical antipsychotics can cause a range of adverse effects, both acute and long-term. These may include:

Extrapyramidal Symptoms (EPS): This includes symptoms like Parkinsonism, dystonia, and akathisia. EPS can be distressing and may lead to medication non-compliance.

Tardive Dyskinesia: This is a potentially irreversible condition characterized by repetitive, involuntary movements of the face, limbs, and trunk.

Neuroleptic Malignant Syndrome (NMS): A rare but life-threatening reaction to antipsychotic drugs characterized by high fever, muscle rigidity, altered mental status, and autonomic dysfunction.

Sedation: Typical antipsychotics can cause drowsiness and impair cognitive and psychomotor function.

Anticholinergic Effects: Dry mouth, constipation, and blurred vision are common side effects.

Weight Gain: Some antipsychotics may lead to significant weight gain.

Hyperprolactinemia: Elevated levels of the hormone prolactin can lead to sexual and reproductive issues.

Atypical Antipsychotics (Second-generation antipsychotics):

Mechanism of Action:

Atypical antipsychotics have a broader mechanism of action compared to typical antipsychotics. They primarily work by blocking the dopamine D2 receptors like typical antipsychotics, but they also affect serotonin (5-HT) receptors, particularly 5-HT2A receptors. By affecting both dopamine and serotonin transmission, they can alleviate both positive and negative symptoms of schizophrenia.

Pharmacokinetics:

The pharmacokinetics of atypical antipsychotics can vary among individual drugs. They are generally well-absorbed after oral administration and have varying half-lives. Many atypical antipsychotics are extensively metabolized in the liver, and their metabolites can be pharmacologically active. Excretion primarily occurs through urine.

Therapeutic Uses:

Atypical antipsychotics are used for the treatment of psychotic disorders, such as schizophrenia and bipolar disorder. They are particularly effective in managing both positive and negative symptoms. In addition to schizophrenia, some atypical antipsychotics are used to treat conditions like major depressive disorder, bipolar depression, and irritability associated with autism spectrum disorders.

Adverse Effects:

Atypical antipsychotics tend to have a more favorable side effect profile compared to typical antipsychotics. However, they are not without side effects, which may include:

Weight Gain: Many atypical antipsychotics are associated with weight gain and may increase the risk of obesity and related conditions.

Metabolic Effects: Increased risk of metabolic issues, including diabetes and dyslipidemia.

Orthostatic Hypotension: Some individuals may experience low blood pressure when changing positions.

Sedation: Drowsiness and somnolence can occur, although it is usually less severe than with typical antipsychotics.

Extrapyramidal Symptoms (EPS): Although less common than with typical antipsychotics, EPS can still occur.

Hyperprolactinemia: Some atypical antipsychotics may increase prolactin levels but typically to a lesser extent than typical antipsychotics.

QT Interval Prolongation: Some drugs in this class may affect the heart's electrical activity, potentially leading to heart rhythm abnormalities.

Agents used in the treatment of anxiety

List of some common drugs and classes of drugs used in the treatment of anxiety disorders:

Selective Serotonin Reuptake Inhibitors (SSRIs):
- Sertraline (Zoloft)
- Escitalopram (Lexapro)
- Fluoxetine (Prozac)
- Paroxetine (Paxil)

Serotonin-Norepinephrine Reuptake Inhibitors (SNRIs):
- Venlafaxine (Effexor)
- Duloxetine (Cymbalta)
- Benzodiazepines:
- Alprazolam (Xanax)
- Lorazepam (Ativan)
- Diazepam (Valium)
- Clonazepam (Klonopin)

Buspirone (Buspar): A non-benzodiazepine anxiolytic.

Beta-Blockers: Sometimes used for specific anxiety-related symptoms.
- Propranolol (Inderal)
- Atenolol (Tenormin)

Tricyclic Antidepressants: While less commonly used for anxiety, they may be prescribed in certain cases.
- Amitriptyline
- Imipramine (Tofranil)

Monoamine Oxidase Inhibitors (MAOIs): Reserved for cases unresponsive to other treatments due to dietary restrictions and drug interactions.

- Phenelzine (Nardil)
- Tranylcypromine (Parnate)
- Pregabalin (Lyrica): Often used for generalized anxiety disorder.

Hydroxyzine (Vistaril): An antihistamine that can have sedative effects and is sometimes used for anxiety.

Antipsychotic Medications: In some cases, atypical antipsychotics are prescribed to manage severe anxiety symptoms.

- Aripiprazole (Abilify)
- Olanzapine (Zyprexa)

Selective Serotonin Reuptake Inhibitors (SSRIs):

Mechanism of Action:

Selective Serotonin Reuptake Inhibitors (SSRIs) work by increasing the levels of serotonin (a neurotransmitter) in the brain. They do this by blocking the reuptake of serotonin in the synapses, which are the gaps between nerve cells. This leads to increased serotonin availability and improved communication between nerve cells, which can help regulate mood and emotional states.

Pharmacokinetics:

Absorption: SSRIs are well absorbed in the gastrointestinal tract, with varying degrees of bioavailability.

Distribution: They are highly protein-bound, primarily to albumin.

Metabolism: SSRIs are extensively metabolized in the liver, primarily by the cytochrome P450 enzymes, especially the CYP2D6 and CYP3A4 subtypes.

Elimination: They are mainly excreted in the urine as metabolites.

Therapeutic Uses:

Major Depressive Disorder (MDD): SSRIs are commonly used as a first-line treatment for depression.

Generalized Anxiety Disorder (GAD): They can help manage symptoms of anxiety.

Panic Disorder: SSRIs are effective in reducing the frequency and intensity of panic attacks.

Obsessive-Compulsive Disorder (OCD): These medications are often prescribed to reduce obsessions and compulsions.

Social Anxiety Disorder (SAD): SSRIs can alleviate symptoms of social anxiety.

Post-Traumatic Stress Disorder (PTSD): They are used to manage symptoms of PTSD.

Premenstrual Dysphoric Disorder (PMDD): SSRIs can help with severe PMS symptoms.

Adverse Effects:

Nausea and Gastrointestinal Distress: Common side effects include nausea, diarrhea, and upset stomach.

Insomnia: SSRIs can disrupt sleep patterns, leading to difficulty falling asleep or staying asleep.

Sexual Dysfunction: This may include reduced libido, difficulty achieving or maintaining an erection, and difficulty achieving orgasm.

Weight Changes: Some people experience weight gain or weight loss.

Serotonin Syndrome: In rare cases, excessive serotonin buildup can lead to this serious condition, characterized by symptoms like high fever, agitation, increased reflexes, tremors, and confusion.

AUTACOIDS ANTAGONISTS

An organic substance, such as a hormone, produced in one part of organism and transported by the blood or lymph to another part of the organism where it exerts a physiologic effect on that part.

AUTACOID The word autacoid comes from the Greek: "autos (self) & " akos (medicinal agent, or remedy)

INTRODUCTION: Histamine, serotonin, prostaglandins, & some vasoactive peptides belong to a group of compounds called Autacoids.

They all have the common feature of being formed by the tissues on which they act so they function as local hormones

The Autacoids also differ from circulating hormones in that they are produced by many tissues rather than in specific endocrine glands.

TYPES: The important Autacoids include:

- Histamine,
- Hydroxytryptamine (5-HT, serotonin),
- Prostaglandins,
- Leukotrienes, and
- Kinins.

HISTAMINE Histamine (Beta-aminoethyl-imidazole) is formed from decarboxylation of Imidazole ring containing amino acid histidine. Histamine is a basic amine, stored in mast cell and basophil granules, and secreted when C3a and C5a interact with specific membrane receptors or when antigen interacts with cell-fixed immunoglobulin E. Histamine plays a central role in immediate hypersensitivity (Type 1) and allergic responses. The actions of histamine on bronchial smooth muscle and blood vessels account for many of the symptoms of the allergic response.

In addition, certain clinically useful drugs can act directly on mast cells to release histamine, thereby explaining some of their untoward effects. Histamine has a major role in the regulation of gastric acid secretion and also modulates neurotransmitter release. Stimulation of IgE receptors also activates phospholipase A2 (PLA2), leading to the production of a host of mediators, including platelet-activating factor (PAF) and metabolites of arachidonic acid. Leukotriene D4, which 2 is generated in this way, is a potent contractor of the smooth muscle of the bronchial tree. Kinins also are generated during some allergic responses. Thus the mast cell secretes a variety of inflammatory mediators in addition to histamine, each contributing to the major symptoms of the allergic response. Epinephrine and related drugs that act through b2 adrenergic receptors increase cellular cyclic AMP and thereby inhibit the secretory activities of mast cells. So are given in anaphylactic shock treatment. However, the beneficial effects of b adrenergic agonists in allergic states such as asthma are due mainly to their relaxant effect on bronchial smooth muscle. Cromolyn or Cromoglicate sodium is used clinically because it inhibits the release of mediators from mast and other cells in the lung. Drug which release histamine: Tubocurarine, succinylcholine, morphine, Polymyxin B, bacitracin, Vancomycin-induced "red-man syndrome" involving upper body and facial flushing and hypotension may be mediated through histamine release. Bradykinin is a poor histamine releaser, whereas kallidin (Lys-bradykinin) and substance P, with more positively charged amino acids, are more active.

- Histamine produces effects by acting on H1, H2 or H3 (and possibly H4) receptors on target cells.
- The main actions in humans are: o Stimulation of gastric secretion (H2) o Contraction of most smooth muscle, except blood vessels (H1) o Cardiac stimulation (H2) o Vasodilatation (H1) o Increased vascular permeability (H1).

Injected intradermally, histamine causes the 'triple response': reddening (local vasodilatation), weal (direct action on blood vessels) and flare (from an 'axon' reflex in sensory nerves releasing a peptide mediator).

The main pathophysiological roles of histamine are: o as a stimulant of gastric acid secretion (treated with H2-receptor antagonists) o as a mediator of type I hypersensitivity reactions such as urticaria and hay fever (treated with H1- receptor antagonists).

H3 receptors occur at presynaptic sites and inhibit the release of a variety of neurotransmitters. 3 H1 antagonists

A. Sedating H1 antagonists (1 st generation antihistaminics)

1. **Chlorpheniramine , Clemastine**
2. **Diphenhydramine**- Mainly used as a mild hypnotic, also show significant antimuscarinic effects
3. **Cyproheptadine** - Used also for migraine due to additional 5-hydroxytryptamine antagonist activity
4. **Promethazine**- Also used for motion sickness, Used for anaesthetic premedication to prevent post- operative vomiting, , weak blockade at α1 adrenoceptors
5. **Hydroxyzine** – used also to treat anxiety
6. **Alimemazine**- Used for premedication
7. **Doxylamine, Triprolidine** - Mainly used as an ingredient of proprietary decongestant and other medicines B. Non-sedating H1 antagonists

Second generation antihistaminics

Second-generation antihistamines, also known as non-sedating antihistamines, are a class of drugs used to treat allergic conditions such as hay fever (allergic rhinitis), hives (urticaria), and other allergic reactions. They work by blocking the action of histamine, a chemical released by the immune system during an allergic response, thereby reducing allergy symptoms. Unlike first-generation antihistamines, second-generation antihistamines have a reduced ability to cross the blood-brain barrier, leading to fewer side effects such as drowsiness and sedation. Some commonly used second-generation antihistamines include:

Second-generation antihistamines, also known as non-sedating antihistamines, are a class of drugs used to treat allergic conditions such as hay fever (allergic rhinitis), hives (urticaria), and other allergic reactions. They work by blocking the action of histamine, a chemical released by the immune system during an allergic response, thereby reducing allergy symptoms. Unlike first-generation antihistamines, second-generation antihistamines have a reduced ability to cross the blood-brain barrier, leading to fewer side effects such as drowsiness and sedation. Some commonly used second-generation antihistamines include:

1. **Loratadine (Claritin):** Loratadine is an over-the-counter antihistamine used to relieve allergy symptoms like sneezing, runny nose, itching, and watery eyes.
2. **Cetirizine (Zyrtec):** Cetirizine is available both over-the-counter and by prescription. It is used for the relief of seasonal and perennial allergic rhinitis and chronic urticaria (hives).
3. **Fexofenadine (Allegra):** Fexofenadine is available both over-the-counter and by prescription. It is used for the treatment of seasonal allergic rhinitis and chronic idiopathic urticaria.
4. **Desloratadine (Clarinex):** Desloratadine is a prescription antihistamine used to treat allergies such as hay fever and hives.
5. **Levocetirizine (Xyzal):** Levocetirizine is a prescription antihistamine used to treat seasonal and perennial allergic rhinitis and chronic urticaria.

Second-generation antihistamines are generally well-tolerated and have a lower risk of causing sedation compared to first-generation antihistamines. They are usually preferred for long-term use in managing chronic allergies due to their favorable side-effect profile. However, individual responses to medications can vary, so it is essential to consult with a healthcare professional before starting any new medication, especially if you have underlying medical conditions or are taking other medications.

Some important drugs:

I. Antihistaminic which increases the appetite and weight gain: **Buclizine**

II. (used for underweight children), **Cyproheptadine, Astimazol**

III. Appetite suppressant While the adnergic drugs called anorectics like **Fenfluramine and Desfluramine** is appetite suppressant.

IV. Local anaesthetic property: **Mepyramine** also have local anaesthetic property also or membrane stabilizing activity (antiarrythimic)

V. Cinnarizine: is drug choice for vertigo, it is antihistaminic, anticholinergic, anti-5- HT and vasodilator It inhibits vestibular sensory nuclei, post-rotatary labyrinthine refluxes by reducing the calcium influx from endolymph into vestibular sensory cells.

VI. Diphenhydramine is generally combined with Thecolic acid to reduce the sedative effect of diphenhydramine.

H2 blockers: are used to treat ulcers and includes the drug like **cimetidine, ranitidine** etc.

EICOSANOIDS

Inflammation induces damage to cell membranes, prompting leukocytes to release lysosomal enzymes. This leads to the liberation of arachidonic acid from precursor compounds, which then undergoes synthesis to produce various eicosanoids.

Among the arachidonate metabolism pathways, the cyclooxygenase (COX) pathway is responsible for generating prostaglandins. These prostaglandins exert diverse effects on blood vessels, nerve endings, and cells involved in the inflammatory process. The discovery of two cyclooxygenase isoforms, COX-1 and COX-2, has shaped our understanding. COX-1 is typically constitutive and plays a role in maintaining homeostasis, while COX-2 is induced during inflammation and facilitates the inflammatory response.

Based on this understanding, highly selective COX-2 inhibitors have been developed and introduced to the market with the assumption that their selectivity would make them safer compared to nonselective COX-1 inhibitors. The goal was to achieve similar effectiveness in treating inflammation without the potential adverse effects associated with nonselective COX-1 inhibition.

In the lipoxygenase pathway of arachidonate metabolism, leukotrienes are produced. These leukotrienes have a strong chemotactic effect on eosinophils, neutrophils, and macrophages, and they also promote bronchoconstriction and changes in vascular permeability.

Moreover, during tissue injury, various substances are released at the site, including kinins, neuropeptides, and histamine. Additionally, complement components, cytokines, and other products of leukocytes and platelets are released. Stimulation of neutrophil membranes results in the generation of oxygen-derived free radicals, which can contribute to further tissue damage.

The superoxide anion is produced when molecular oxygen undergoes reduction, and it can trigger the generation of other reactive molecules like hydrogen peroxide and hydroxyl radicals. When these reactive species interact with arachidonic acid, they lead to the production of chemotactic substances, which perpetuate the inflammatory process.

In mammals, arachidonic acid (5, 8, 11, 14-eicosatetraenoic acid) serves as the primary precursor for eicosanoid synthesis. This 20-carbon unsaturated fatty acid contains four double bonds, which explains the terms "eicosa" (referring to the 20 carbon atoms) and "tetraenoic" (referring to the four double bonds). Arachidonic acid plays a critical role in the production of various bioactive compounds involved in inflammation and other physiological processes.

In most cell types, arachidonic acid is esterified in the phospholipid pool, resulting in low concentrations of the free acid. The main eicosanoids synthesized from arachidonic acid include prostaglandins, thromboxanes, and leukotrienes. Additionally, other derivatives of arachidonate, such as lipoxins, are also generated.

The liberation of arachidonate is typically the initial and rate-limiting step in eicosanoid synthesis. This liberation can occur through a one-step process or a two-step process, both of which are facilitated by the enzyme phospholipase A2 (PLA2). This enzyme plays a key role in releasing arachidonic acid from phospholipids, thus initiating the production of eicosanoids.

Various enzymes play a role in eicosanoid synthesis, with the cytosolic phospholipase A2 (cPLA2) being the most important due to its strict regulation. This enzyme not only produces arachidonic acid (the precursor of eicosanoids) but also lysoglycerylphosphorylcholine (lyso-PAF), which gives rise to platelet-activating factor (PAF), another inflammatory mediator. Once arachidonic acid is released, it can be metabolized through different pathways, some of which include:

- Fatty acid cyclo-oxygenase (COX): This pathway involves two main isoforms, COX-1 and COX-2, which transform arachidonic acid into prostaglandins and thromboxanes. Prostaglandins and thromboxanes play crucial roles in various physiological processes and inflammatory responses.
- Lipoxygenases: This pathway comprises several subtypes of enzymes that synthesize leukotrienes, lipoxins, and other related compounds. Leukotrienes, for instance, have potent chemotactic effects and contribute to the

inflammatory process, while lipoxins are involved in regulating inflammation and promoting the resolution of inflammation.

Overall, the metabolism of free arachidonic acid through these pathways leads to the production of a diverse array of eicosanoids, each with specific functions in inflammation and various physiological processes.

PHARMACOLOGY OF DRUGS ACTING ON RENAL SYSTEM: ANTIDIURETICS

An antidiuretic is a substance that aids in water retention within the body, preventing the kidneys and bladder from eliminating water too rapidly. Medicines with antidiuretic properties are utilized to treat conditions such as bed-wetting, incontinence, and similar disorders.

Specifically, antidiuretic drugs are employed to decrease urine volume, particularly in cases of diabetes insipidus (DI), a condition characterized by excessive thirst and the production of large amounts of dilute urine.

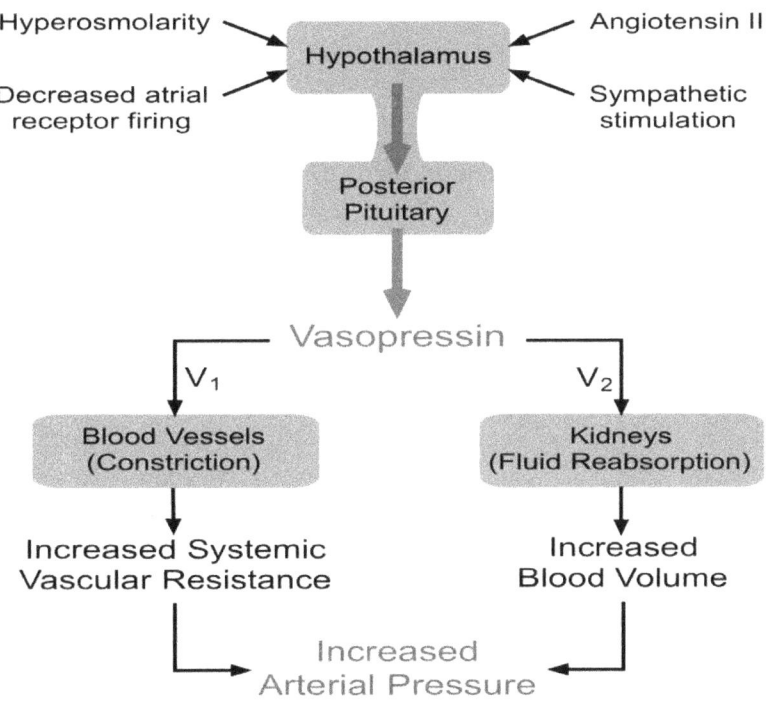

VASOPRESSIN

- **Structure & Synthesis of ADH**

Vasopressin, commonly known as antidiuretic hormone (ADH), is a neurohypophysial hormone present in most mammals. In many species, it consists of arginine and is also referred to as Arginine Vasopressin (AVP) or Argipressin.

The hormone is initially synthesized as a pre-prohormone and then undergoes processing to form a nonapeptide, which is a peptide composed of nine amino acids.).

The amino acid sequence of arginine vasopressin (argipressin) is Cys-Tyr-Phe-Gln-Asn-Cys-Pro-Arg-Gly-NH2. In this sequence, the cysteine residues form a disulfide bond, and the C-terminus of the sequence is converted to a primary amide.

Lysine vasopressin (Lypressin) is a related hormone found in pigs and some other animals, which has a lysine in place of the arginine as the eighth amino acid in the sequence. On the other hand, arginine vasopressin is the form found in humans.

> **Function**

Vasopressin has two primary functions:

1. Water Retention: It helps the body retain water by reducing the amount of water excreted through urine. This is achieved by increasing the reabsorption of water in the kidneys, leading to a decrease in urine volume.
2. Vasoconstriction: Vasopressin acts as a vasoconstrictor, causing the blood vessels to narrow. This constriction of blood vessels leads to an increase in blood pressure.

Lysine vasopressin (LVP) or lypressin is a similar substance found in pigs, and it serves the same functions as vasopressin. Lypressin is also used in human therapy for similar purposes.

Vasopressin is released in response to reductions in plasma volume and increases in plasma osmolality. When the body senses decreased blood volume or increased blood concentration (osmolality), it triggers the release of vasopressin to conserve water and maintain proper fluid balance.

Higher concentrations of antidiuretic hormone (vasopressin) cause arterioles to constrict, resulting in increased arterial pressure. This mechanism contributes to maintaining blood pressure within a normal range.

Additionally, the secretion of antidiuretic hormone is stimulated by decreases in blood pressure and volume, ensuring that the body responds appropriately to changes in fluid levels and maintains homeostasis.

1. Kidney:

Vasopressin exerts three main effects:

- Increased Water Permeability: It enhances the water permeability of cells in the distal convoluted tubule and collecting duct of the kidneys. This allows for increased water reabsorption, resulting in the excretion of more concentrated urine, a process known as antidiuresis.
- Increased Calcium Concentration: Vasopressin causes episodic release of calcium from intracellular stores in the collecting duct cells, leading to an increase in the concentration of calcium within these cells.
- Acute Increase in Sodium Absorption: It acutely increases the absorption of sodium across the ascending loop of Henle in the kidney. This contributes to the counter-current multiplication mechanism, aiding in proper water reabsorption later in the distal tubule and collecting duct.

These effects of vasopressin collectively play a crucial role in regulating water balance and concentration of urine in the body, ensuring proper fluid homeostasis.

2. Cardiovascular system

Vasopressin has the additional effect of increasing peripheral vascular resistance, which means it causes vasoconstriction in the peripheral blood vessels. As a result of this vasoconstriction, the arterial blood pressure is elevated.

In healthy individuals, this effect of vasopressin is relatively minor. However, in cases of hypovolemic shock, such as during severe hemorrhage (excessive bleeding), this vasoconstrictive effect becomes a crucial compensatory mechanism to help restore blood pressure. By constricting the blood vessels, vasopressin helps maintain blood flow to essential organs and tissues, ensuring that adequate oxygen and nutrients are delivered even during states of low blood volume. This response is essential for the body to cope with life-threatening situations and prevent further deterioration in blood pressure and perfusion to vital organs.

3. Central nervous system

Vasopressin released within the brain has various actions:

- Circadian Rhythm: Vasopressin is released in a circadian rhythm by neurons of the suprachiasmatic nucleus, helping to regulate the body's internal clock and daily biological rhythms.
- Involvement in Aggression, Blood Pressure, and Temperature Regulation: Vasopressin released from centrally projecting hypothalamic neurons plays a role in regulating aggression, blood pressure, and temperature in the body.
- Modulation of Corticosteroid Release: Vasopressin likely acts in conjunction with Corticotropin-Releasing Hormone (CRH) to modulate the release of corticosteroids from the adrenal gland in response to stress. This interaction is especially significant during pregnancy and lactation in mammals.
- Analgesic Effects: Recent evidence suggests that vasopressin may have analgesic (pain-relieving) effects. These analgesic effects of vasopressin appear to be dependent on both stress levels and sex, meaning that the response varies based on the individual's stress levels and gender.

Use of vasopressin

Vasopressin has been used for various medical purposes over the past 50 years, including:

- ✓ Treating Neurogenic Diabetes Insipidus: Vasopressin is used to manage central diabetes insipidus, a condition characterized by excessive thirst and the production of large amounts of dilute urine due to insufficient antidiuretic hormone (ADH) production.
- ✓ Reducing Bleeding and Blood Transfusions during Burn Wound Excision: Vasopressin has been employed to decrease bleeding and the need for blood transfusions during burn wound excision procedures.
- ✓ Treating Upper Gastrointestinal Hemorrhage: Vasopressin is used to manage severe upper gastrointestinal bleeding secondary to conditions like hemorrhagic gastritis.

- ✓ Treating Severe Hematuria: Vasopressin has shown effectiveness in treating cases of severe hematuria, where there is abnormal blood loss in the urine.
- ✓ Reducing Blood Loss and Preventing Intraoperative Hypotension during Liver Transplant: Vasopressin is utilized to minimize blood loss and prevent intraoperative hypotension during liver transplant surgeries.
- ✓ Treating Refractory Bleeding after Uterine Myoma Resection: Vasopressin is used in cases of persistent and difficult-to-control bleeding after uterine myoma resection.
- ✓ Use of Vasopressin in Cardiac Arrest: Vasopressin is sometimes used as an alternative to adrenaline (epinephrine) in the treatment of cardiac arrest to improve blood flow and circulation.
- ✓ Uterine Contraction: Vasopressin acts on oxytocin receptors to cause uterine contractions. In the nonpregnant and early pregnancy uterus, vasopressin is equally potent as oxytocin in inducing contractions. However, at term (near the end of pregnancy), the uterus becomes more sensitive to oxytocin selectively.

These diverse applications of vasopressin highlight its therapeutic potential in various medical conditions, particularly those involving bleeding, blood pressure regulation, and uterine contractions.

Von Willebrand's Disease is the most common inherited bleeding disorder in humans, characterized by a deficiency or abnormality of von Willebrand factor (vWF). This protein plays a vital role in blood clotting, and its deficiency can lead to prolonged bleeding and difficulties in forming blood clots after injuries or surgeries. Treatment involves various approaches to manage bleeding episodes effectively.

ADH (Vasopressin) receptors

These are G protein coupled cell membrane receptors; two subtypes V1 and V2

1. V1-receptors:

The receptors for vasopressin (V1 receptors) are further classified into two subtypes:

1. V1a Receptors: These are found on vascular and other smooth muscles, platelets, liver, and other tissues. When activated, they function through the phospholipase and diacylglycerol (DAG) pathway, leading to the release of calcium ions (Ca^{2+}) from intracellular stores. This, in turn, causes vasoconstriction (narrowing of blood vessels), contraction of visceral smooth

muscles, glycogenolysis (conversion of glycogen to glucose), and the release of adrenocorticotropic hormone (ACTH) from the anterior pituitary gland.

2. **V1b Receptors:** These receptors are localized to the anterior pituitary gland. Their activation also involves the phospholipase and DAG pathway, leading to the release of calcium ions (Ca2+) from intracellular stores. This process further stimulates the release of ACTH from the anterior pituitary.

Both subtypes of V1 receptors' actions are amplified by the increased influx of calcium ions (Ca2+) through calcium channels, which enhances the physiological effects mentioned above.

2. V2 Receptors: The V1 receptors are primarily located in various tissues, including vascular and smooth muscle cells, platelets, and the liver. When activated, they initiate the phospholipase and diacylglycerol (DAG) pathway, leading to vasoconstriction, smooth muscle contraction, glycogenolysis, and ACTH release from the anterior pituitary gland. V2 receptors are mainly found in the collecting duct cells of the kidney, regulating water permeability through cAMP production. Additionally, vasodilatory V2 receptors are present in blood vessels. V2 receptors are more sensitive to ADH than V1 receptors, responding to lower concentrations of the hormone.

Here is the table 3 with ADH (Vasopressin) receptors, their locations, and main functions:

ADH (Vasopressin) Receptor	Location	Main Function
V1A Receptor	Smooth muscle cells	Vasoconstriction (narrowing of blood vessels)
		Regulation of blood pressure and vascular tone
		Stimulation of hepatic glycogenolysis (glucose release)
V1B Receptor	Anterior pituitary gland	Modulation of hormone release, including ACTH
		Involved in the stress response and cortisol production
V2 Receptor	Kidney (collecting duct)	Increases water reabsorption from urine

| | | Concentration of urine and conservation of body water |
| | | Helps maintain body fluid balance and osmolarity |

Mechanism of Action of Vasopressin

Vasopressin is a peptide hormone formed in the hypothalamus, then transported via axons to, and released from, the posterior pituitary.

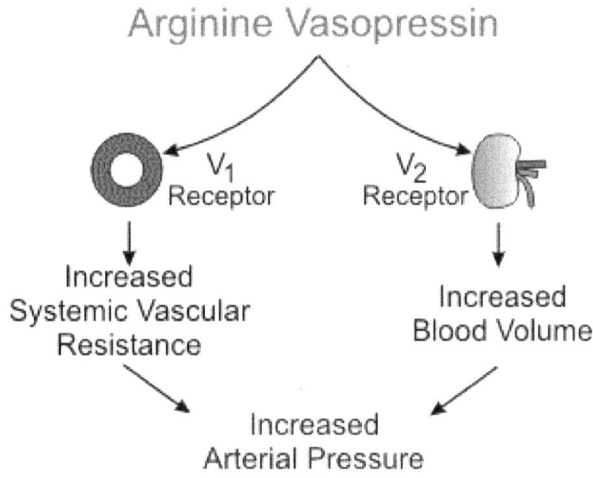

There are several mechanisms regulating the release of AVP.

- Hypovolemia, as occurs during hemorrhage, results in a decrease in atrial pressure. Specialized stretch receptors within the atrial walls and large veins (cardiopulmonary baroreceptors) entering the atria decrease their firing rate when there is a fall in atrial pressure. Atrial receptor firing normally inhibits the release of AVP by the posterior pituitary. With hypovolemia or decreased central venous pressure, the decreased firing of atrial stretch receptors leads to an increase in AVP release.

- Hypothalamic osmoreceptors sense extracellular osmolarity and stimulate AVP release when osmolarity rises, as occurs with dehydration. Finally, angiotensin II receptors located in a region of the hypothalamus regulate AVP release – an increase in **angiotensin II** simulates AVP release.

- AVP has two principal sites of action: the kidney and blood vessels. The most important physiological action of AVP is to increase water reabsorption in the kidneys by increasing water permeability in the collecting duct, thereby permitting the formation of more concentrated urine. This is the antidiuretic effect of AVP and it acts through vasopressin type 2 receptors (V2) coupled to adenylyl cyclase.

- AVP also constricts arterial blood vessels by binding to V1 receptors, which are coupled to the G-protein couple receptor.

Drugs which increase vasopressin release.	Drugs which increase vasopressin release
Vincristine, Cyclophosphamide, Tricyclics, Nicotine Barbiturates, Adrenaline, High dose opiate	Ethanol, Phenytoin, Corticosteroids, Haloperidol, Phenergan (promethazine), Low dose opiate

❖ Disease States

- The most common disease related to antidiuretic hormone is diabetes insipidus. This condition can arise from either of four situations:

i. Hypothalamic ("central") diabetes insipidus results from a deficiency in secretion of antidiuretic hormone from the posterior pituitary. Causes of this disease include head trauma, and infections or tumors involving the hypothalamus.

ii. Nephrogenic diabetes insipidus occurs when the kidney is unable to respond to antidiuretic hormone. Most commonly, this results from some type of renal disease, but mutations in the ADH receptor gene or in the gene encoding aquaporin-2 have also been demonstrated in affected humans.

iii. Dipsogenic diabetes insipidus or primary polydipsia results from excessive intake of fluids as opposed to deficiency of arginine vasopressin. It may be due to a defect or damage to the thirst mechanism, located in the hypothalamus or due to mental illness.

iv. Gestational diabetes insipidus occurs only during pregnancy and the postpartum period. During pregnancy, women produce vasopressinase in the placenta, which breaks down ADH. Gestational DI is thought to occur with excessive production and/or impaired clearance of vasopressinase.

Aquaporins

- Aquaporins also called water channels, are integral membrane proteins

- Aquaporins are "**the plumbing system for cells**," Every cell is primarily water. "But the water doesn't just sit in the cell, it moves through it in a very organized way. The process occurs rapidly in tissues that have these **aquaporins or water channels**."

- There are thirteen known types of aquaporins in mammals, and four of these are located in the kidney.

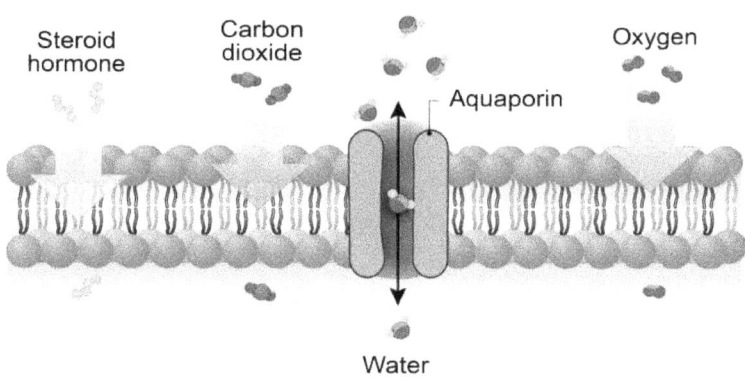

Fig. 7 Aquaporins

NOTE BY

• **ENURESIS:** incontinence may be a continual inability to manage evacuation. Involuntary evacuation is additionally referred to as enuresis. Its two varieties are as under

(i) Diurnal incontinence daytime wetting.

(ii) Nocturnal incontinence, conjointly known as bedwetting

- **INVOLUNTARY URINATION**: Urinary incontinence (UI), conjointly famous as involuntary evacuation, is any escape of weewee

- NOCTURNAL incontinence

- Nocturnal incontinence is involuntary evacuation that happens in the dark whereas sleeping.

- There square measure 3 types of enuresis:

i. Primary nocturnal incontinence: Primary nocturnal enuresis (PNE) is that the most typical style of bedwetting. It happens due to psychosocial issues for youngsters and their oldsters. errhine factors could embody organic process delay, genetic influence, difficulties in waking and diminished nighttime secretion of vasoconstrictor.

ii. Secondary nocturnal incontinence: Secondary enuresis happens when a patient goes through Associate in Nursing extended amount of xerotes in the dark (roughly six months or more) so reverts to nighttime time wetting. Secondary incontinence may be caused by emotional stress or a medical condition, like a bladder infection.

iii. Psychological nocturnal enuresis: Its is continual evacuation into bed or garments, occurring doubly per week or additional for a minimum of 3 consecutive months in a very kid of a minimum of five years older and undue to either a drug facet impact or a medical condition.

- **Causes of bedwetting square measure**
  - Neurological-developmental delay
  - Genetics
  - **Alcohol consumption**: Drinking alcohol will increase weewee production, inhibits anti-diuretic endocrine production, decreases awareness, will increase somnolence and causes impulsive choices.
  - Insufficient production of internal secretion, or short response to internal secretion, results in Associate in Nursing overrun of weewee.
  - Caffeine will increase weewee production.
  - Chronic constipation will cause bed wetting. Once the bowels square measure full, it will place pressure on the bladder.

The most common of that may be a tract infection.

Sleep symptom stemming from Associate in Nursing higher airway obstruction has been associated with bedwetting.

Snoring and enlarged tonsils.

Sleepwalking will result in bedwetting.

Nocturnal incontinence may be the presenting symptom of diabetes, classically related to nephrosis, polydipsia, and polyphagia; weight loss and lethargy. Serious sleeping

- Somnambulation

- It's conjointly referred to as sleeping or sleepwalking, may be a development of combined sleep and wakefulness.

- It's classified as a disorder happiness to the parasomnia family.

- Somnambulation happens throughout slow wave sleep stage in a very state of low consciousness.

- These activities may be as benign as sitting up in bed, walking to a rest room, and cleansing, or as dangerous

as cooking, driving, violent gestures, grabbing at hallucinated objects or maybe putting to death.

- **PARASOMNIAS**

- Parasomnias (para = abnormal or incorrect; somnia = Sleep) square measure a cluster of sleep disorders in that Something goes awry with a person's sleep cycle.

- There square measure 5 common types' parasomnias: (i) somnambulation, (ii) REM sleep behavior disorder, (iii)

Nightmares (bad dreams), (iv) Night terrors, (v) Teeth grinding.

DRUGS AFFECTING RESPIRATORY SYSTEM

Drugs affecting the respiratory system are divided into 5 groups:

1. Respiratory stimulants;

2. Drugs used to treat cough (Antitussives);

3. Expectorants;

4. Bronchodilators (drugs used to treat asthma);

5. Drugs used to control pulmonary edema.

Respiratory stimulants Respiratory stimulants are classified according to corresponding influence on the sides of the CNS and by type mechanism of action. Frequency and depth of breathing are regulated by breathing center. Respiratory stimulants excite breathing centre and than increase lung ventilation and gas metabolism, oxygen content and decrease carbonic acid level. They increase metabolism products excretion, stimulate oxidative processes and acid-based equilibrium. They may increase arterial pressure by excitation of vessel moving centre and increase of haemodinamics.

Below is a table 4 listing some common drugs that affect the respiratory system, along with their respective actions and uses:

Drug Name	Action	Uses
Bronchodilators	Relax bronchial smooth muscles	Asthma, Chronic Obstructive Pulmonary Disease (COPD)
Corticosteroids	Reduce inflammation in airways	Asthma, Allergic Rhinitis, COPD, Inflammatory Lung Conditions

Antihistamines	Block histamine receptors	Allergic Rhinitis, Upper Respiratory Allergies
Expectorants	Promote mucus clearance	Cough with Mucus
Antitussives	Suppress cough reflex	Dry, Non-productive Cough
Mucolytics	Break down thick mucus	Respiratory Conditions with Thick Mucus
Leukotriene Inhibitors	Block leukotrienes, reduce inflammation	Asthma, Allergic Rhinitis
Long-acting Beta-2 Agonists	Relax bronchial smooth muscles	Asthma, COPD
Inhaled Corticosteroids	Reduce inflammation in airways	Asthma, COPD
Oxygen Therapy	Provides supplemental oxygen	Hypoxia, Respiratory Failure
Anticholinergics	Block cholinergic receptors	COPD, Asthma (as an adjunct therapy)
Antibiotics	Treat respiratory infections	Bacterial Respiratory Infections

Table 4 some common drugs that affect the respiratory system, along with their respective actions and uses

The respiratory stimulants may be divided:

- Drugs which mainly influence cortex (coffeinum-natrii benzoas);
- Drugs which mainly influence medulla oblongata (Aethimizolum, Camphora, Sulfocamphocainum, Cordiaminum, Bemegridum);
- Drugs which mainly influence spinal cord (Strychnini nitras). They are also divided into:
- Drugs of direct action on respiratory centre (Coffeini natrii benzoas, Aethimizolum, Bemegridum);
- Drugs of reflexive action (Lobelini Hydrochloride, Cytitonum, solutio Ammonii causticum);
- Drugs of mixed action (Carbogenum (95-93 % O_2, 5-7 % CO_2), Cordiaminum, Camphora, Sulfocamphocainum).

Bemegridum is not used in Ukraine.

Aethimizolum is a derivative of dicarbone acid, blocks phosphodiesterase accumulates cAMP, increases frequency and depth of respiration, heart rate, dilutes bronchial muscles. It may stimulates formation of glucocorticoids, has antinflammative immunomodulative action, increases tonus of cardiac and skeletal muscles. The drug has a sedative action. It is used in overdosage or poisoning with narcotic drugs for general anesthesia, alcohol, hypnotic drugs, in the case of asphyxia of newborns.

Adverse effects may be the following: dyspepsia, disturbance of sleep, anxiety, dizziness.

Camphora is terpene ketone from silver fir oil which is half synthetical. **Sulfocamphocainum** is a derivative of sulfocamphoral acid and Novocain and may be administered intravenously, subcutaneously, intramuscularly. These drugs stimulate respiratory and cardiomotor centres. Camphora stimulates heart. Camphora and sulfocamphocainum are used in cases of poisoning by narcotic drugs, carbonate oxydum in asphyxia, cardiac insufficiency.

Adverse effects. Camphora may cause irritation and sulfocamphocainum – idiosyncrasy. Cytitonum, and lobelini hydrochloride stimulate N-cholinoreceptors located in the CNS, carotide glomerules, and adrenal medulla. They are used as respiratory stimulants very seldom, more often in case of poisoning with carbonate oxide. Solutio Ammonii causticum irritates receptors of nose mucosa and then respiratory centre in case of dizziness byreflex. Carbogen excites vasomotor centre, narrows peripheral vessels. It is used in case of poisoning by narcotic agents, carbonic oxide, asphyxia, different diseases with insufficiency of 162 respiratory system.

Antitussives

Antitussines are divided into:

1. Drugs of central action:

a) Opioides – codeine phosphus, aethylmorphini hydrochloridus which suppress the cough reflex by depressing a medullary cough centre;

b) Nonopioide drugs – glaucini hydrochloride, oxeladini cytras, and synecodum.

2. Drugs of peripheral action: Libexinum which has broncholytical and local anesthetic effect. Falimint has also antimicrobial effect. The antitussives are used in case of dry cough.

Expectorants

These drugs are divided into:

1. Bronchosecretor drugs which assist liquid mucose expelling;

2. Mucolytics which melt mucose. Bronchosecretor drugs are classified as:

a) **Drugs of reflector action** - infusum herbal Thermopsidis, decoctum radicis Althaeae, Mucaltinum; They irritate receptor of stomach mucosa, increase secretion of bronchial glands, contractility of epithelium and muscles and help mucus expelling. Infusum herbae Thermopsidis also excites respiratory centre. Decoctum radicis Althaeae and Mucaltinum have covering effect.

b) **Resorbtive action;** Kalii iodidum which excretes through glands, melts mucus and stimulates secretion. Natrii hydrocarbonate changes pH to base district and stimulatessecretion.

3. There are mixed expectorants

Mycolytics are divided into:

a) **Proteolytic enzymes;** They tear peptide connections, change physicochemical properties of mucus. There are such drugs as Trypsini crystallisatum, **Chymotrypsiin crystallisatum, Desoxyribonucleasa**, Ribonucleasa. Two last drugs change depolimerisation of nucleonic acids

b) **Synthetic mucolytics** – Acetylcysteinum, Carbocysteinum; 163 They have sulfhydryl groups that tear disulfide connections and help mocose expelling. Besides this acetylcysteinum is antioxidant, cardioprotector, antidotum of paracetamolum.

c) **Synthetic mucolytics** that increase synthesis of surfoctntum – Bromhexinum, Ambroxolum; These drugs also have thiogroups which open mucoproteins disulfide groups, reducing the viscosity of mucose. They will not provoke bronchospasm in patients with bronchial asthma.

d) **Drugs of surfactant** which change surfactant content in alveols – Alveofact, Exosurf.

Bronchodilators

Airflow obstruction in asthma is due to the inflammation of bronchial wall, contraction of bronchial smooth muscle, increased mucus secretion causing shortness of breath and makes respiration difficult. An asthmatic attack may be precipitated by inhalation of allergens (dust, perfume, pollen, animal) which interact with mast cells coated with immunoglobuline E, generated in response to a previous exposene to allergen. The mast cells release mediators such as histamine, leukotrienes, and hemotaxic factors, which promote bronchiolar spasm and mucosal thickening from edema and cellular infiltration. Many asthmatic attacks are not rereluted to a recent exposure to allergen, but rather reflect bronchial hyperactivity of unknown origin which is somehow related to inflammation of the airway mucosa. The symptoms of asthma may be effectively treated by several drugs, but no one of the agents provide a cure for this obstructive lung disease.

There are five groups of the bronchodilators:

1. Adrenergic agents; The adrenergic agents with beta activity are the drugs of choice for mild intermitted asthma. These potent bronchodilators relax airway smooth muscle and inhibit the release of substances from mast cells which cause bronchoconstriction. The most common agents are beta2- **adrenomimetics – salbutamolum, fenoterolum, terbutalinum, formoterolum, salmeterolum, and clenbuterolum. Salbutamolum, fenoterolum, terbutalinum** are the drugs of short duration (4-5 hours) and are used for prevention and treatment of asthma attacks. Salmeterolum, clenbuterolum, and formoterolum have a prolonged action and are used for prevention of asthma attacks. Beta1,2-adrenomimetics (isadrinum and orciprenalini sulfas) are used seldom.In acute attack 164 adrenalini hydrochloridum and ephedrini hydrochloridum may be administered. Stimulation of beta2-adrenoreceptors leads to increasing of cAMP – concentration, decreasing of Ca^{2+} ion concentration, relaxation, stabilization of basophilic cell, and membranoprotection action.

2. M-cholinoblockers are less effective-Ipratropii bromidum, Atropini sulfas, Platyphyllini hydrotartras, Methacinum are used as bronchodilators. They increase cGMP concentration, decrease Ca^{2+} ions concentration lead to smooth muscle relaxation. Inhaled ipratropii bromidum a quaternary derivative of atropine sulfas is useful in patients unable to take adrenergic agonists.

3. **Myotropic broncholytics (Xantines).** When asthmatic symptoms cannot be controlled with adrenergic agents addition of the methylxanthine derivatives may be appropriate. Myotropic bronchodilatators relieve airflow obstruction in acute asthma and decrease the symptoms of chronic diseases. The drugs are well absorbed in gastrointestinal tract and there are several sustained release preparations. There are euphyllinum, theophyllinum in that group. Overdoses of the drugs may cause seizures or arrhythmias.

4. **Nonsteroid inflammatory drugs**. Cromolyn–sodium is an effective prophylactic agent which stabilizes the membrane of most cells and prevents mediator release by blocking calcium gate. The drug is not useful in managing in acute asthmatic attack. For use in asthma cromolyn-sodium is administerd as inhalation of a microfine powder or as an aerosolized solution. Because it is poorly absorbed only minor adverse effects are associated with it. Pretreatment with cromolyn–sodium blocks allergeninduced and exercise–induced bronchoconstriction. Cromolyn–sodium is also useful in reducing the symptoms of allergic rhinitis. Not all patients respond to a cromolyn–sodium therapy, but those who do respond to the treatment show improvement which is roughly equal to the improvement obtained from main tename euphyllinum or theophyllinum therapy. Nedochromylum–natrium is more effective. It also decreases content of leucotriens and stimulates neuropetideC.

Ketotiphenum decreases histamine release and blocks H1-histamine receptors. It is used for prophylactic of bronchospasm. It is possible to use other antihistaminic drugs (diprazinum, suprastinum and others). 165

5. **Corticosteroids.** Prednisolonum, dexamethasonum, triamcinolonum, budesonidum, flunisolidum, fluticasonum, and beclomethasonum are used for prevention of bronchial asthma attacks.

Drugs used to control pulmonary edema:

I. Drugs decreasing hydrostatic pressure in lung vessels.

1. Natrii nitroprussidum and organic nitrates (nitroglycerinum, isosorbidi dinitras);

2. Ganlioblockers (pentaminum, benzohexonium, hygronium);

3. Broncholytics (euphyllinum);

4. Drugs with alpha – blocking properties (aminazinum, diprazinum);

5. Tranquilisers (diazepamum);

6. Opioid analgetics (morphini hydrochloridum);

7. Narcotic analgetics with neuroleptics (phentanylum + droperidolum or haloperidolum);

8. Corticosteroids (prednisolonum and others).

II. Drugs improving heart contractility.

1. Cardiac glycosides (corglyconum, digoxinum, strophanthinum);

2. Nonglycosides cardiotonics (dophaminum, dobutaminum), may be administered with the APE inhibitors;

III. Drugs decreasing circulating blood volume.

1. Loop diuretics – furosemidum, torasemidum.

2. Osmotic diuretics in the conditions of tolerancy to furosemidum (mannitolum, mannitum, urea pura rarely)

IV. Drugs restoring normal bronchial and bronchiols passage transforming gas into alveols in liquid (alcohol).

DRUGS ACTING ON GASTROINTESTINAL TRACT

Digestants These drugs are used to promote digestion of food as a replacement therapy in condition of their deficiency specially in atrophic gastritis, gastric carcinoma, pernicious anaemia or pancreatic insufficiency etc. Various proteolytic (pepsin, papain), lipolytic (lipases) and amylolytic (diastase and takadiastase) enzymes are used in combination as appetite stimulants and health tonics. Dilute hydrochloric acid (HCl) is advocated in severe achlorhydria. These are beneficial only when deficiency of these is marked, otherwise their routine use is irrational and unwarranted.

Digestants in Gastric Dysfunction

1. **Hydrochloric acid**- 5 to 10 ml of 10% HCl, diluted further in 100-200 ml of water may be sipped with a straw (to avoid direct contact with teeth) during meals. When taken in sufficient quantity HCl will help in enhancing the activity of pepsin (both of endogenous/exogenous source) and may prevent bacterial growth in stomach during achlorhydria.

2. **Pepsin**- it may be used with HCl in condition of deficiency. Dose- 20 to 100 mg/day in divided doses contained in various marketed enzyme preparations.

3. **Papain**- raw papaya contains papain which has got proteolytic activity. Dose- 30-60 mg/day as advocated in different enzyme preparations.

Digestants in Pancreatic Insufficiency

1. **Diastase/takadiastase**- They are amylolytic enzymes obtained from fungus Aspergillus oryzae. Dose- Takadiastase-150-160 mg/day and diastase-around 20 mg/day in various marketed preparations.

2. **Pancreatin-** it is a mixture of various pancreatic enzymes like amylase, trypsin and lipase, generally obtained from hog/pig pancreas. It reduces fecal fat and nitrogen content. It should be given by enteric coated capsule to prevent its own digestion in stomach by pepsin. It can produce adverse reactions like nausea, diarrhea and uric acid renal stones. Dose-150-250 mg/day in various marketed preparations with simethicone (25 mg) or tauroglycocholate (50 mg).

Emetics and Antiemetics Drugs:- Vomiting or emesis is a protective mechanism which leads to expulsion of harmful substances from the upper gastrointestinal tract (GIT). It involves the active participation of vomiting centre (VC) present in the medulla oblongata either through direct afferent input to it or via chemoreceptor trigger zone (**CTZ**) and nucleus tractus solitarius (NTS) present in area postrema. Impulses from the higher cortical centres due to unpleasant sight, smell or thought, pain, emotional factors and increase in intracranial pressure etc. may induce vomiting. Similarly impulses via cerebellum arising from vestibular apparatus (inner ear) stimulation either by frequent change in body motion or its stimulation by ototoxic drugs like aminoglycosides can also induce vomiting. Both NTS and CTZ act as relay station for VC and receive impulses from GIT, heart, testis, throat, and other viscera through vagus and sympathetic nerves. Afferents from fauces run through NTS to the VC. CTZ which lies outside the blood brain barrier is accessible to circulating drugs (cytotoxic drugs, levodopa, apomorphine, digitalis, ergot alkaloids etc.), mediators (5-Hydroxytryptamine released by platelets or inflamed site), toxins (infection), 2 hormones (oestrogen etc.), radiation etc. The motor pathways activated by VC lead to relaxation of cardiac end of stomach and contraction of diaphragm and abdominal muscles to increase the intragastric pressure allowing the gastric contents to expel out. Vomiting generally follows the inhibition of gastric motility believed to be mediated through dopamine receptor (DA2). VC contains mainly cholinergic muscarinic (M) receptors, whereas vestibular apparatus has both M and histamine-1 (H1) receptors. CTZ and NTS have variety of receptors like M, H1, DA2 and 5-hydroxytryptamine-3 (5-HT3). Enkephalins are also implicated in mediation of vomiting acting possibly at δ (CTZ) or μ (vomiting centre) opoid receptors. Substance P acting at neurokinin – 1 receptor in CTZ may also play a role. Table 1shows the pathways for either stimulation of relay centers (CTZ, NTS) or VC or both and the types of receptors present which lead to vomiting.

Fig 1: Receptors and pathways involved in stimulation of NTS, CTZ and Vomiting Centre and choice of drugs

- Sight, smell, taste, pain,   -Motion sickness, -Ototoxic drug -

-Raised intracranial pressure   -Emotional factors

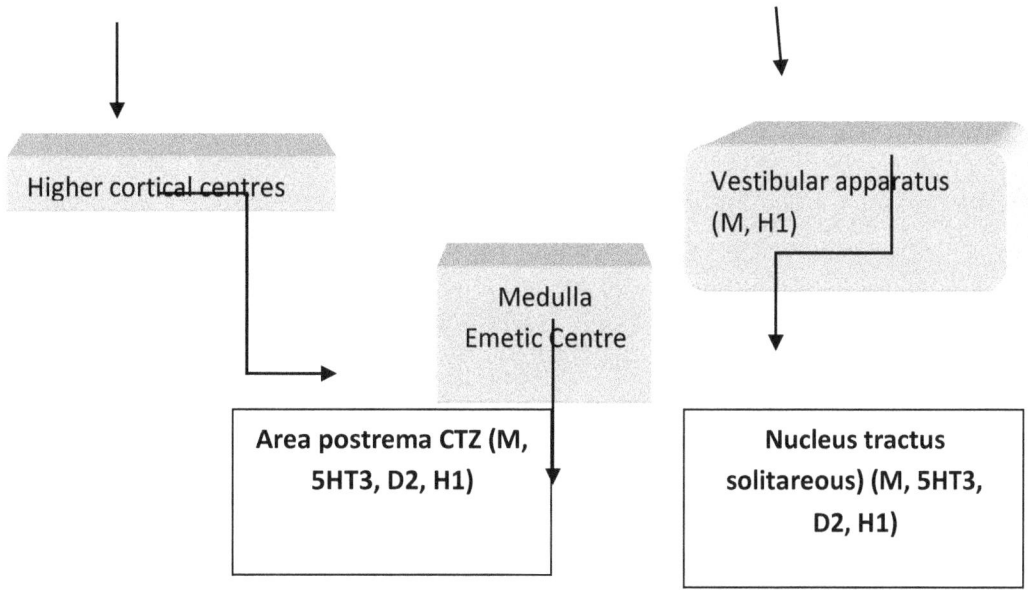

i) Blood borne emetics (5-HT, cytotoxic drugs, levodopa, VOMITING apomorphine, digitalis etc)

- ii) Release of emetogenic agents- 5HT, Prostanoids and free radicals in g.i.t. stimulating nerves to CTZ and NTS
- iii) Radiation
- iv) Infection (toxin)

Emetics

Emetics are drugs used to evoke vomiting when a toxic substance has been swallowed. They may either act directly (*apomorphine*) or reflexly on CTZ (*Ipecacuanha*). Apomorphine is a semisynthetic derivative acting as dopaminergic agonist on CTZ. Apomorphine (6mg) induces vomiting within 5-10 minutes when injected intramuscularly or subcutaneously. *Ipecacuanha* containing emetine is used as syrup (15-20 ml in adults). Copper sulphate, 3powdered mustard suspension or oil or strong salt solution can also be used in emergency. They act through stimulation of receptors in stomach. Elimination of respiratory depression should be made before using the above drugs. Emetics are contraindicated in poisoning of any corrosive (danger of perforation), CNS stimulant (precipitation of convulsion), kerosene (aspiration pneumonia due to low viscosity), morphine or phenothiazine (emetics are ineffective) and in unconscious patients (danger of aspiration due to absence of laryngeal reflex).

Antiemetics

These drugs are generally employed for the treatment of nausea or vomiting induced by motion sickness, morning sickness, gastrointestinal disturbance, postoperative emesis, cytotoxic drug or radiation-evoked emesis. Variety of drugs, having different chemical and pharmacological profiles is useful antiemetic agents. They are classified as follows:

1. **Antimuscarinic** – Hyoscine, dicyclomine etc.

2. **H1-antihistaminics** – Promethazine, Diphenhydramine dimenhydrinate, cyclizine, Meclizine, cinnarizine etc.

3. **Neuroleptics** – Chlorpromazine, prochlorperazine, haloperidol, droperidol etc.

4. **Prokinetics-** Metoclopramide, domperidone, cisapride etc.

5. **5HT3 antagonist**– Ondansetron, granisetron, bemesetron, renzapride, zacopride etc.

6. **Miscellaneous** – Dexamethasone, benzodiazepine, Cannabinoids etc.

1. Antimuscarinic drugs : Hyosine is used for prophylaxis as well as for the treatment of motion sickness. Administered in 0.2 – 0.4 mg dose either oral or intramuscular, it has got short duration of antiemetic action. It blocks the cholinergic pathway from vestibular apparatus to vomiting centre but is ineffective against drugs acting directly on CTZ. It produces side effects like drowsiness, dryness of mouth, blurring of vision and retention of urine. **Dyclomine** is used in prophylaxis of motion sickness and morning sickness in oral doses of 10-20 mg per day.

2. H1-antihistaminics: The use of H1-antihistaminics is based on their central anticholinergic, antihistaminic and sedative properties. They are effective in vomiting due to motion sickness, Meniere's disease, pregnancy, uremia and postoperative emesis. Peripheral antimuscarinic action is also important for antiemetic effect. H1-antihistaminics have little or no activity against substances inducing vomiting by acting directly on CTZ though they are effective in motion sickness and substances active locally in stomach to induce vomiting. These should be avoided in first trimester of pregnancy to avoid any foetal damage. Promethazine theoclate (avomine, 25 mg Tab.) is especially promoted as antiemetic. It produces sedation and dryness of mouth. Cyclizine and meclizine are long acting antihistaminics and mainly used for sea sickness (24 hrs). Cinnarazine is recently introduced anti-vertigo drug which has in addition to H1-blocking property also inhibits influx of calcium from endolymph into the vestibular sensory cells which mediates labyrinthine reflexes. Drug used for motion sickness should be given half to one hour before journey.

3. Neuroleptics : They are potent drugs blocking D2 receptors in CTZ. These are mainly used in chemotherapy-, post-anaesthetic-, disease-, malignancy- and radiation sickness-induced vomiting and vomiting in hyperemesis gravidarum. **They are not effective in motion sickness. Phenothiazines-** the antiemetic dose of phenothiazines such as chlorpromazine, prochlorperazine is about 20-30% of their antipsychotic dosage whereas the dose for perphenazine is similar. They can cause significant degree of sedation and acute muscle dystonia in children specially girls. Haloperidol and droperidol are mainly used to control postoperative vomiting and vomiting in patients on cancer chemotherapy.

4. Prokinetic drugs: They promote gastroduodenal peristalsis and speed gastric emptying. Metoclopramide is chemically related to procainamide. It increases gastric peristalsis while relaxing pylorus and 1st part of duodenum. This is independent of vagal innervation but their action is more prominent when vagus is intact. On CTZ, it acts by selective blocking of D2 receptor inhibiting apomorphine-induced vomiting. At the periphery it enhances Ach release causing gastric prokinetic effect and enhancing lower oesophageal sphincter tone. Prokinetic action of metoclopramide is blocked by atropine. At high doses it acts as 5HT3 antagonist. It is rapidly absorbed orally, enters brain, crosses placenta and is secreted in milk. It causes sedation, dizziness, diarrhea and muscle dystonia. On long term use it can cause **parkinsonism, galactorrhoea and gynaecomastia.** It should not be used to augment lactation because it is secreted in milk. It hastens absorption of many drugs like aspirin and diazepam (facilitating gastric emptying). It reduces the extent of absorption of digoxin by allowing less time for it.

Bioavailability of cimetidine is also reduced. By blocking dopamine receptors in basal ganglia, it abolishes therapeutic effect of levodopa. **It is used mainly as antiemetic, gastrokinetic in dyspepsia and GERD.** It is administered in a dose of 10 mg three times a day orally (po) or intramuscularly (im). In children the dose is 0.25 to 0.5 mg/kg (po and im). It is available as 10 mg Tablet (Perinorm), 5 mg / 5 ml syrup, 10 mg/2 ml injection for oral or im use.

Domperidone is D2 antagonist and is a lower efficacy antiemetic and prokinetic agent. Prokinetic action is not blocked by atropine. It crosses into CNS poorly (cf. CTZ which is outside the Blood Brain Barrier). Extra pyramidal side effects are rare but hyperprolactinemia can occur. Its efficacy is lower than metoclopramide. It is orally absorbed with bioavailability of 15% (1st pass metabolism) and its t½ is 7.5 hrs. It can cause cardiac arrhythmias on rapid I.V. injection (10-40 mg Tab.). Administered with levodopa and bromocriptine it counteracts their dose limiting emetic action without affecting the therapeutic effect in parkinsonism. Dose is 10-40 mg, three times a day in adult and 0.3 to 0.6 mg/kg in children.

Cisapride is a prokinetic agent which resembles metoclopramide but has **no central depressant or D2 antagonist or any action on CTZ**. Its action is blocked by atropine. Cisapride stimulates 5HT4 receptors and increases cAMP activity and releases Ach from myentric plexus. Oral bioavailability is 33% and is primarily inactivated through liver. Its t½ is 10 hrs and dose should be reduced in liver diseases. It can cause arrhythmias with macrolides and imidazoles. Its main use is in gastroesophageal reflux disease. Dose is 10-20 mg, three times a day in adult.

5. 5HT3 antagonist : Ondansetron and granisetron have been introduced for the control of cytotoxic-induced vomiting. Renzapride, zacopride, bemasetron, and tropisetron are recently introduced 5HT3 antagonist used to prevent nausea and vomiting after cancer chemotherapy. Ondansetron- It blocks the depolarizing action of 5HT through 5HT3 receptors or vagal afferents in the GIT as well as in NTS and CTZ. It blocks the emetogenic impulses both of central and peripheral origin. Its oral bioavailability is 60-70% (1st pass metabolism). Its t ½ is 3-5 hrs and duration of action varies from 4-12 hrs. It should be given half an hour before chemotherapeutic infusion as slow i.v. injection.

6. Miscellaneous: Cannabinoids- Nabilone, a synthetic cannabinol derivative is found to be effective against CTZ-stimulated vomiting. Its effect is blocked by naloxone. It is given orally. Its plasma half life is 120 min and is excreted both in urine and faeces. Unwanted effects include drowsiness, dry mouth, dizziness and postural hypotension. Steroids like dexamethasone and methylprednisolone have antiemetic activity in high doses probably through inhibition of prostaglandin synthesis. Neurokinin-1 antagonists (**Vofopitant, GR 05171**) suppressing substance P can also act as an effective antiemetic agent.

Choice of antiemetic drugs

• **H1 receptor antagonist** – Cyclizine – motion sickness – Promethazine – severe morning sickness of pregnancy and space motion sickness — Cinnarizine – Motion sickness, vestibular disorder (meniere's disease)

• **Muscarinic receptors antagonists** — Hyosine – Motion sickness

• **D2 receptor antagonists** — Phenothiazines – Emesis induced by uraemia, radiation, viral gastroenteritis and severe morning sickness of pregnancy. — Metoclopromide – Emesis induced by uraemia, radiation, GI disorder, cytotoxic agents

• **5HT3 antagonist** — Ondansetron - Emesis induced by cytotoxic anti cancer drugs and radiation and postoperative vomiting

• **Cannabinoids** — Nabilone - Emesis induced by cytotoxic anticancer drugs

Pathogenesis: Dyspepsia, in its various forms has been mankind's companion since the advent of bad cooking, overindulgence and anxiety. For several decades, the dictum " no acid-no ulcer" has dominated the pharmacological basis of treatment of ulcer therapy, and the drugs used, reduced acid secretion. However, in 40-70% patients of duodenal ulcer (DU), acid secretion is within normal limits, whereas in gastric ulcer (GU) acid secretion is either normal or below normal. Patients of **Zollinger-Ellison syndrome**, characterized by abnormally high acid secretion, show minimal incidence of peptic ulceration. It is therefore, apparent that peptic ulceration is not solely induced by offensive acid and pepsin secretion. Breakdown of mucosal resistance which constitute mucin bicarbonate secretion, phospholipids layer and tight junctions, cell proliferation, prostaglandins, epidermal growth factors, mucosal blood flow etc. have got an important role to play in ulcerogenesis Fig. 1). In a broad sense, ulcers are thought to be due to an imbalance between aggressive and defensive mucosal factors. The treatment of peptic ulcer disease is thus, directed towards strengthening the mucosal defensive factors rather reducing acid-pepsin activity.

Histamine H2-receptor antagonists

• Histamine-2 (H2) receptor antagonists prevent acid reflux by competitively blocking the H2 receptors of the parietal cells in the stomach, thus reducing gastric acid secretion.

• Example: cimetidine (Tagamet®), ranitidine (Zantac®), famotidine (Pepcid®), nizatidine (Axid®)

Antacids

• Substances that promote ulcer healing by neutralizing HCl and reducing pepsin activity.

• Antacids can interact with other drugs

• by adsorption or binding of the other drugs (decreasing oral absorption of bound drug)

• by increasing stomach pH (causing a decrease in absorption of certain drugs)

• by increasing urinary pH (inhibiting elimination of drugs that are weak bases).

• Antacid use in animals has decreased due to difficulty of administration and the introduction of histamine-2 blockers

Mucosal Protective Drugs

• Mucosal protective drugs, also known as pepsin inhibitors, are typified by the drug sucralfate (Carafate®).

• Sucralfate is a chemical derivative of sucrose that is nonabsorbable and combines with protein to form an adherent substance that covers the ulcer and protects it from stomach acid and pepsin.

• Sucralfate comes in 1-g tablets, and its only side effect is constipation.

- Because sucralfate binds to ulcers in an acid environment, it should not be given at the same times as H2 receptor antagonists.

Prostaglandin Analogs

- Prostaglandin analogs appear to suppress gastric secretions and increase mucus production in the GI tract.

- An example of a prostaglandin analog is misoprostol (Cytotec®)

- An oral tablet that is usually given to animals taking nonsteroidal anti-inflammatory drugs (NSAIDs).

Proton Pump Inhibitors

- Proton pump inhibitors are drugs that bind irreversibly to the H+-K+-ATPase enzyme on the surface of parietal cells of the stomach.

- This inhibits hydrogen ion transport into the stomach so that the cell cannot secrete HCl.

- When this enzyme is blocked, acid production is decreased, and this allows the stomach and esophagus to heal.

Regimen	Duration, days	Drugs used	Notes
Triple therapy	7–14	PPI (standard dose) bid, amoxicillin 1 g bid and clarithromycin 0.5 g bid	First line therapy in areas with low clarithromycin resistance
Sequential therapy	10	1st 5 days: PPI (standard dose) bid and amoxicillin 1 g bid; 2nd 5 days: metronidazole 0.5 g bid and clarithromycin 0.5 g bid	First line therapy

Drugs That Promote Upper Gastrointestinal Motility

Motility stimulants

•Prokinetic agents increase the motility of parts of the GI tract to enhance movement of material through it.

•Parasympathomimetic agents, dopaminergic antogonists, and serotonergic agents may act as prokinetics.

Dopaminergic Antagonists

•Dopaminergic antagonists stimulate gastroesophageal sphincter, stomach, and intestinal motility by sensitizing tissues to the action of the neurotransmitter acetylcholine.

• Side effects are behavioral in nature.

• Examples of dopaminergic antagonists include metoclopramide (Reglan®) and domperidone (Motilium®).

Serotonergic Agents

• Serotonergic agents stimulate motility of the gastroesophageal sphincter, stomach, small intestine, and colon.

•Cisapride (Propulsid®), used for the treatment of constipation, gastroesophageal reflux, and ileus.

• Side effects may include diarrhea, megacolon, and abdominal pain

ANTIDIARRHOEAL AGENTS:-

•Diarrhoea is the frequent passage of liquid faeces, and this is generally accompanied by abdominal cramps and sometimes nausea and vomiting.

•It may be viewed as a physiological mechanism for rapidly ridding the gut of poisonous or irritating substances.

•There are numerous causes, including underlying disease, infection, toxins and even anxiety

•It may also arise as a side effect of drug or radiation therapy. During an episode of diarrhoea, there is an increase in the motility of GIT, accompanied by an increased secretion coupled with a decreased absorption of fluid, which leads to a loss of electrolytes (particularly Na^+) and water. Cholera toxins and some other bacterial toxins produce a profound increase in electrolyte and fluid secretion by irreversibly activating the guanine nucleotide regulatory proteins that couple the surface receptors of the mucosal cells to adenylate cyclase

There are three approaches to the treatment of severe acute diarrhoea:

• Maintenance of fluid and electrolyte balance •use of anti-infective agents

• use of spasmolytic or other antidiarrhoeal agents.

The maintenance of fluid and electrolyte balance by means of oral rehydration is the first priority, and wider application of this cheap and simple remedy could save the lives of many infants in the developing world. Many patients require no other treatment. In the ileum, as in parts of the nephron, there is cotransport of Na^+ and glucose across the epithelial cell. The presence of glucose (and some amino acids) therefore enhances Na^+ absorption and thus water uptake. Preparations of sodium chloride and glucose for oral rehydration are available in powder form, ready to be dissolved in water before use.

DRUGS USED IN GASTROINTESTINAL DISORDERS

Drugs stimulating appetite are amara tinctura Absinthii, plantaglucidum, and others which irritate mouth mucosa receptors. **Anorexigenic drugs** include as main central serotonin agonist sibutramidum (meridia) which oppresses hunger centre and peripheral drug orlistatum (xenicalum) inhibiting lipase.

Other drugs which inhibit hunger center:

- **inhibit cateholamine system** – phepranonum, desopimonum, and mazindolum;
- **inhibit serotonine system** – phenphluraminum. Drugs which increase gastrointestinal motility Decreased gastrointestinal motility can be result of a systemic disease, intrinsic gastrointestinal disorders or medication. **These drugs are classified as:**
  - **M-Cholinomimetic drugs** – aceclidinum;
  - **Anticholinestherase drugs** – proserinum, pyridostigmini bromidum, and distigmini bromidum;
  - **Prokinetics** – metoclopramidum (cerucalum), cisapridum (propulsid), and tegaserodum (Zelnorm). Metoclopramidum is central dopamine antagonist resulting in increased gastric contraction, enhanced gastric emptying and small lower transit, cause antiemetic effect. Peripherally it stimulates the release of intrinsic postganglionic stores of acetylcholine and sensitizises the gastric smooth muscle to muscarinic stimulation. It can decrease the acid reflux into the esophagus.

Therapeutic uses: Metoclopramidum is used in patients with diabetic, postoperative idiopathic gastroparesis, in lower esophagus sphincter pressure, as antiemetic drug.

Adverse effects are fatigue, insomnia, after motor coordination, Parkinsonian side effects, acute dystonic reactions. Cisapridum and teguserodum are serotonin-4 (5HT4) receptor agonist, facilitute the release of acetylcholine. Cathartics stimulate afferent nerves to initiate a reflex increase in gut motility. Plant cathartics are divided into oils (oleum Ricini) and the drugs consisting of anthraguinone derivatives. Oils. **Oleum Ricini** is a bean oil which is hydrolyzed in the gut to ricinoleic acid and glicerinum. The ricinoleic acid acts on the ileum and colon to induce an increased fluid secretion and colonic contraction. It is used in acute obstipation. Anthraguinone derivatives (drugs of senna, rhei, aloe etc). They biotransform to emetinum and acidum chrisophanicum which irritate receptors of colon rather than on the ileum, produce evacuation in 8-10 hours.

The main drugs are **senadexinum**, fun sena.

Synthetic drugs - isapheninum, bisacodylum, natrii picosulfas (guttalax), also irritate colon receptors and are used as antaguinone derivatives in chronic obstipation.

Osmotic catharthics (magnesii sulfas) increase Lumen osmolarity, irritate intestine receptors. They are used in intoxication.

Osmotic laxatives (e.g. lactulose, sorbitolum are purely absorbed, and draw additional fluid into gastrointestinal tract, increase lumen osmolarity.

Oleum Vasselini, Oleum Amygdalarum are stool softeners. Methylcellulosa, laminaridum are bulk-forming laxatives.

Drugs that decrease gastrointestinal motility are divided into:

- M-Cholinoblockers: atropine sulfas, platyphyllini hydrotartras, and methacinum;
- Spasmolytics: papaverini hydrochloridum, no-spanum, mibeverinum;
- Drugs for treating diarrhea;
- Agonists opioid receptors – loperamidum, domperidonum;
- Silicate drugs – enterosgelum, silix; smekta, kaopectate;

- Microlial drugs;
- Lactobacteries – lactobacterium;
- Sugarmiceties – enterolum;
- Probiotics – chylack, linex;
- Others – colybacterinum, lactobacterinum, biosporinum etc.

Loperamide is agonist of opioid receptor. It protects against diarrhea, reduces the daily fecal volume, and decreases intestinal fluid and electrolyte loss.

Adverse effects: Abdominal pain, distention, constipation, dry mouth, hypersensitivity, nausea, vomiting, dizziness.

Emetic drugs are divided into:

Drugs of central action – apomorphini hydrochloridum acting on the hemoreceptor trigger zone connecting to the emetic centre through the fasciculus solitarius;

Antiemetics are classified into:

- Antihistamines – diprazinum (pipolfenum);
- Dophamine receptors blockers – metoclopramidum (cerucalum), domperidonum (motilium), thiethylperatinum (forecanum);
- Anticholinergics - scopolamini hydrobromidi (Aeronum);
- SHT3 receptor agonists – ondausetronum (Zofranum), granicetronum (Kytrilum), tropisetronum (Novobanum);
- Drugs increasing stomach secretion. These group of drugs is divided into:
- Diagnostic drugs – pentagastrinum;
- Drugs of replacing therapy – acidum hydrochloricum dilutum, pepsinum, succus gastricus naturalis that indicate in hypoacidic, anacidic gastritis, achylia. Polyenzyme drugs such as Pancreatinum, Festalum, Panzinorm forte, Mezym forte are used when secretion of stomach glands, pancreas, bile secretion are diminished.

Drugs that decrease gastric acid secretion are divided into:

Here's the classification of drugs that decrease gastric acid secretion in table 5:

Drug Class	Mechanism of Action	Examples
Proton Pump Inhibitors (PPIs)	Inhibit gastric proton pump (H+/K+ ATPase), reducing acid secretion.	Omeprazole, Lansoprazole, Esomeprazole
H2 Blockers (H2 Antagonists)	Block histamine-2 receptors in the stomach, reducing histamine-induced acid production.	Ranitidine, Famotidine, Cimetidine
Antacids	Neutralize existing stomach acid, providing quick but short-term relief.	Tums, Maalox, Rolaids
Mucosal Protective Agents	Enhance the protective mucous layer in the stomach, reducing damage from stomach acid.	Sucralfate, Misoprostol
Prostaglandin Analog	Increases mucus production in the stomach while inhibiting acid production.	Misoprostol
Reflux Suppressants	Reduce acid reflux into the esophagus.	Alginate-based medications

here is a classification of gastroprotective drugs in table form:

Class	Mechanism of Action	Examples
Mucosal Protective Agents	Enhance the protective mucous layer in the stomach to reduce damage caused by stomach acid.	Sucralfate
Prostaglandin Analog	Increase mucus production in the stomach and inhibit acid production.	Misoprostol

Antacids	Neutralize existing stomach acid, providing quick but short-term relief from acidity and heartburn.	Tums, Maalox, Rolaids, etc.
Reflux Suppressants	Reduce acid reflux into the esophagus, often used to treat gastroesophageal reflux disease (GERD). Some formulations are based on alginates.	Alginate-based medications

Omeprazole is the prototype of the benzimidazole sulfoxide prodrugs that diffuse across the gastric parietal cell cytoplasm, where they are protonated. It binds to parietal cell H +, K +-ATPase, inhibiting secretion of hydrogen ions into the gastric lumen.

➢ Omeprazole is unstable in acid and is formulated in gelatin capsules. It is metabolized in the liver and excreted in the bile and urine.

➢ By irreversibly inhibiting parietal cell H +, K+-ATPase and preventing the secretion of hydrogen ions into the gastric lumen, the drug appears to be more effective than ranitidinum for treatment of patients with gastroesophageal reflux. It has antihelicobacter effect.

➢ Omeprazole inhibits the oxidative metabolism of phenytoin, diazepam, and other drugs.

➢ Although the incidence of adverse effects is low, toxicologic studies using high doses of Omeprazole have demonstrated gastric carcinoid tumors in rats. Intense acid suppression leads to increased gastrin secretion, which has a trophic effect on gastric mucosa. Other proton pump inhibitors have the same pharmacodynamics. Rabeprazolum is the most effective. EsOmeprazole, isomer of Omeprazole, has better pharmacokinetics. Antacides interact with the HCL. Some of them are absorbed: Magnesium oxide, **Sodium hydrogen carbonate, Calcium carbonate, and Magnesium trisilicate**. Sodium hydrogen carbonate can cause systemic alkalization, sodium overload formation of heart increasing secretion. Calcium carbonas may induce hypercalciemia and reload increase of gastric secretions. Magnesii oxydum and magnesii hydroxydum may produce osmotic diarrhea and excessive absorption of magnesium in patients with renal failure may result in the CNS toxicity.

Aluminii hydroxidum is association with constipation. Almagel, Maalox and aluminii hydroxidum are not absorbed. Agents that reduce gastric acidity (gastroprotectors)

Gastroprotective drugs aim to increase the stability of the gastric and duodenal mucosa against the harmful effects of gastric acid. These drugs are classified based on their effects on haemopoiesis, particularly erythropoiesis, used to treat anemia. Anemia, characterized by lower-than-normal plasma hemoglobin concentration due to a decrease in red blood cell count or reduced hemoglobin content, can result from various causes such as chronic blood loss, bone marrow abnormalities, increased hemolysis, infections, malignancies, endocrine deficiencies, and other medical conditions.

These drugs can be categorized into those used for hypochromic (iron-deficiency) anemias, hyperchromic anemias, and anemias associated with chronic renal failure.

Drugs for Hypochromic (Iron-Deficiency) Anemias:

Iron preparations come in various forms, including monodrugs and complex drugs for oral and parenteral administration.

- Iron preparations for oral administration include ferrous sulfate (ferri sulfas), ferrous fumarate (ferri fumaras), ferrous gluconate (ferri gluconas), and ferrous chloride (ferri chloridum).
- Iron preparations are primarily in the Fe^{2+} form, as Fe^{3+} may irritate the mucosa. In the stomach, iron is converted into its ionic form.
- In the intestines, Fe^{2+} binds to protein apoherritin to form ferritin complexes, which are then transported into the bloodstream.
- Iron is actively transported as Fe^{2+}. A limited diffusion of Fe^{2+} may occur when it forms complexes with amino acids, vitamins, or food peptides.
- In the bloodstream, Fe^{2+} dissociates and binds with beta1 globulin (transferrin), forming a complex that is transported to the bone marrow or stored in depo tissues like the liver and spleen.
- In the bone marrow, Fe^{2+} is used to synthesize hemoglobin, while in depo tissues, it is stored in complexes with apoferritin as ferritin.

- Iron has various uses, including hemoglobin formation in erythrocytes, hemin (myoglobin) formation, and other non-hemoglobin functions in the body.
- Therapeutic uses: Iron deficiency, hypochromic anemias, chronic hemorrhage, iron malabsorption, pregnancy, and dystrophies.

Adverse effects: Dyspepsia, constipation, tooth darkening, and nausea.

Complex iron drugs include tardiferonum, actiferinum, and ferroplex, among others. Factors like amino acids, riboflavin, peptides, dilute hydrochloric acid, ascorbic acid, biometals (cobalt, magnesium, manganese, gold), and an intact mucosa assist iron absorption. Calcium, antacids, tetracycline, chloramphenicol, and phytates can inhibit iron absorption.

For situations where oral administration is not feasible, there are parenterally administered drugs like Fercovenum and Ferrum Lek, but they can lead to adverse effects such as hypotension, allergic reactions, and nausea.

Drugs for Hyperchromic Anemias:

Cyanocobalamin (Vitamin B12) and folic acid are the primary drugs used in hyperchromic anemias.

Cyanocobalamin is converted into cobalamin, a cofactor for folic acid reductase, and plays a role in purine, pyrimidine, nucleic acid, and protein synthesis.

In cases of cyanocobalamin deficiency, disturbances in bone marrow function may occur, leading to the transformation of erythrocytes into megaloblasts. It is absorbed in pernicious anemia.

Therapeutic uses: Cyanocobalamin is used to treat hyperchromic malignant anemias, pernicious megaloblastic anemia (Addison-Birmer anemia), iron-deficiency anemias, hypoplastic anemias, radiation diseases, neurological disorders, and immune deficiencies.

Adverse effects: Overdose symptoms can include excitement, tachycardia, allergy, increased coagulation, and heartaches.

Folic acid plays a crucial role in purine, pyrimidine, nucleic acid, and amino acid synthesis, normal erythropoiesis, regeneration, leukopoiesis, thrombopoiesis, and immune system activity.

Therapeutic uses: Folic acid is used to treat macrocytic anemias in conditions like lactation, pregnancy, alcoholism, sprue, postoperative anemia, newborns, radiation diseases, and chronic gastric enteritis.

Adverse effects: Concrement formation and B12 deficiency.

III. Drugs used in anaemias due to chronic renal failure

Drugs used in the treatment of anemias due to chronic renal failure (CRF) can be classified into several categories, each with its mechanism of action and associated adverse effects.

Erythropoiesis-Stimulating Agents (ESAs):

Mechanism of Action: ESAs, such as epoetin alfa and darbepoetin alfa, are synthetic forms of erythropoietin. They stimulate the bone marrow to produce more red blood cells.

Adverse Effects: Common side effects include hypertension, headaches, flu-like symptoms, and injection site reactions. More serious risks include pure red cell aplasia (rare), increased risk of thrombosis, and exacerbation of pre-existing hypertension.

Iron Supplementation:

Mechanism of Action: Iron is necessary for hemoglobin synthesis. In CRF patients, iron deficiency is common, and supplements are used to correct this deficiency and improve the effectiveness of ESAs.

Adverse Effects: Adverse effects may include gastrointestinal discomfort, constipation, and iron overload, which can harm organs such as the liver and heart.

Intravenous Iron Preparations:

Mechanism of Action: These preparations deliver iron directly into the bloodstream, rapidly increasing iron levels in patients with chronic renal failure and iron deficiency.

Adverse Effects: Adverse effects may include hypersensitivity reactions (including anaphylaxis), injection site reactions, and gastrointestinal symptoms.

Vitamin B12 and Folate Supplements:

Mechanism of Action: These supplements address anemias associated with vitamin B12 or folate deficiency, which can contribute to anemia in CRF patients.

Adverse Effects: *These supplements are generally well-tolerated, but very high doses can cause side effects.*

Blood Transfusions:

Mechanism of Action: Blood transfusions directly provide red blood cells, raising hemoglobin and hematocrit levels in patients with severe anemia.

Adverse Effects: Risks of transfusions include transfusion reactions (allergic or hemolytic reactions), iron overload from repeated transfusions, and the potential for transmission of infectious diseases (which is minimized through donor screening and testing).

Phosphate Binders:

Mechanism of Action: Phosphate binders, such as sevelamer or calcium-based binders, are used to manage high phosphate levels often seen in CRF. They may indirectly improve anemia by reducing secondary hyperparathyroidism, which can suppress erythropoiesis.

Adverse Effects: Adverse effects may include gastrointestinal disturbances, calcium accumulation in blood vessels and tissues, and interactions with other medications.

ACE Inhibitors and Angiotensin Receptor Blockers (ARBs):

Mechanism of Action: These medications are often used to control blood pressure and mitigate proteinuria in CRF patients. They may help to improve anemia by reducing renal damage and inflammation.

Adverse Effects: Common side effects include dizziness, elevated potassium levels, and kidney function changes. ACE inhibitors can cause a persistent cough.

Antidiarrhoeal Therapy

Dehydration is the most common cause of death in case of diarrhea. So correction of fluid depletion, shock and acidosis are of central importance to all forms of acute diarrhea. Treatment should always be directed according to the underlying cause as most diarrhoea is self limiting. The treatment of diarrhea therefore, consists of correction of dehydration by oral rehydration therapy, maintenance of adequate nutrition and drug therapy which can be either specific against the microbials or non-specific antidiarrhoeal agents.

Antidiarrheal therapy refers to the treatment and management of diarrhea, a condition characterized by frequent, loose, or watery bowel movements. Diarrhea can be caused by various factors, including infections, gastrointestinal disorders, food intolerances, and medications. Antidiarrheal treatments aim to alleviate the symptoms and underlying causes. Here are some common approaches to antidiarrheal therapy:

Oral Rehydration Solution (ORS):

Mechanism of Action: ORS is a mixture of water, salts, and sugar that helps replace lost fluids and electrolytes due to diarrhea. It prevents or treats dehydration associated with diarrhea.

Indications: ORS is recommended for mild to moderate cases of diarrhea, particularly in children and in cases of infectious diarrhea.

Adverse Effects: Generally safe, but improper preparation may lead to incorrect electrolyte balance.

Loperamide (Imodium):

Mechanism of Action: Loperamide is an opioid receptor agonist that acts on the gut to slow down intestinal motility, leading to less frequent and more formed bowel movements.

Indications: Loperamide is used for short-term relief of acute diarrhea and chronic diarrhea associated with conditions like irritable bowel syndrome (IBS).

Adverse Effects: Side effects may include constipation, dizziness, and abdominal discomfort. It should be used with caution in certain conditions, and long-term use should be avoided.

Bismuth Subsalicylate (Pepto-Bismol):

Mechanism of Action: Bismuth subsalicylate has both antimicrobial and anti-inflammatory properties. It can reduce the frequency of diarrhea by acting on the gut lining and inhibiting some bacterial pathogens.

Indications: It is used to relieve symptoms of traveler's diarrhea and mild infectious diarrhea. It can also help manage symptoms of indigestion and heartburn.

Adverse Effects: May cause temporary darkening of the tongue and stool. Should not be used by individuals with aspirin allergies or certain medical conditions.

Antibiotics:

Mechanism of Action: Antibiotics may be used to treat specific bacterial infections that cause diarrhea. They target and eliminate the causative bacteria.

Indications: Antibiotics are reserved for cases of bacterial or parasitic diarrhea when there is evidence of infection. They should only be used under the guidance of a healthcare professional.

Adverse Effects: Antibiotics can have various side effects and should only be used when necessary to avoid antibiotic resistance.

Dietary Modifications:

Mechanism of Action: Avoiding specific food triggers and adopting a bland diet can help reduce irritation and inflammation in the gastrointestinal tract.

Indications: Dietary modifications are typically used to manage chronic conditions like IBS or food intolerances.

Adverse Effects: There are generally no adverse effects associated with dietary changes, but individual tolerance varies.

Underlying Cause Management:

Mechanism of Action: Treating the underlying cause of diarrhea, such as an infection, food intolerance, or medication side effect, is essential in resolving the condition.

Indications: Determined by the specific underlying cause of the diarrhea.

Adverse Effects: Adverse effects depend on the treatment approach used to address the underlying cause.

ANTIMOTILITY AND SPASMOLYTIC AGENTS

Antimotility and spasmolytic agents are a class of drugs that affect the gastrointestinal system by either slowing down or relaxing the muscles of the digestive tract. These drugs are used to treat a variety of conditions, including diarrhea, irritable bowel syndrome (IBS), and other gastrointestinal disorders. Here are some examples of antimotility and spasmolytic agents and their mechanisms of action:

Loperamide (Imodium):

Mechanism of Action: Loperamide is an opioid receptor agonist that acts on the gut to slow down intestinal motility. It reduces the frequency and urgency of bowel movements, making stools less watery.

Indications: Loperamide is used for the short-term relief of acute diarrhea and chronic diarrhea associated with IBS.

Adverse Effects: Side effects may include constipation, dizziness, and abdominal discomfort. It should not be used in cases of bloody diarrhea, high fever, or underlying infections.

Diphenoxylate with Atropine (Lomotil):

Mechanism of Action: Diphenoxylate is an opioid receptor agonist that slows down intestinal motility, while atropine is included to discourage abuse due to its anticholinergic effects.

Indications: Lomotil is used for the treatment of diarrhea.

Adverse Effects: Common side effects include drowsiness, dizziness, and dry mouth. It should be used with caution and only under the guidance of a healthcare provider.

Hyoscyamine (Levsin):

Mechanism of Action: Hyoscyamine is an anticholinergic agent that helps to relax smooth muscle in the gastrointestinal tract. It reduces spasms and can alleviate symptoms of IBS.

Indications: It is used to relieve symptoms of irritable bowel syndrome, as well as other conditions involving gastrointestinal muscle spasms.

Adverse Effects: Side effects may include dry mouth, blurred vision, and dizziness. It should be used under medical supervision.

Dicyclomine (Bentyl):

Mechanism of Action: Dicyclomine is another anticholinergic agent that reduces muscle spasms in the gut, helping to relieve abdominal pain and discomfort.

Indications: It is used to treat symptoms of IBS and other gastrointestinal disorders associated with muscle spasms.

Adverse Effects: Adverse effects can include dry mouth, dizziness, and constipation. It should be used as directed by a healthcare professional.

Peppermint Oil:

Mechanism of Action: Peppermint oil has antispasmodic effects on the gastrointestinal tract, helping to relax smooth muscles and relieve symptoms of IBS.

Indications: It is used as a natural remedy to alleviate abdominal pain, bloating, and spasms in individuals with IBS.

Adverse Effects: Side effects may include heartburn and allergic reactions in some individuals.

These medications are used to manage conditions in which excessive motility and muscle spasms in the gastrointestinal tract lead to symptoms like diarrhea, abdominal pain, and cramps. It's important to use these drugs under the guidance of a healthcare provider, as they may have side effects or interactions with other medications. Additionally, they are typically not recommended for use in cases of severe infectious diarrhea.

Here's a table 6 summarizing common antimotility and spasmolytic agents along with their mechanisms of action:

Drug	Mechanism of Action	Indications	Adverse Effects
Loperamide (Imodium)	Opioid receptor agonist that slows intestinal motility.	Short-term relief of acute diarrhea, chronic diarrhea (associated with IBS).	Constipation, dizziness, abdominal discomfort.
Diphenoxylate with Atropine (Lomotil)	Opioid receptor agonist with atropine to discourage abuse.	Treatment of diarrhea.	Drowsiness, dizziness, dry mouth.
Hyoscyamine (Levsin)	Anticholinergic agent that relaxes smooth GI muscles.	Relief of IBS symptoms, other conditions with GI spasms.	Dry mouth, blurred vision, dizziness.
Dicyclomine (Bentyl)	Anticholinergic agent that reduces GI muscle spasms.	Treatment of IBS and other GI disorders with muscle spasms.	Dry mouth, dizziness, constipation.
Peppermint Oil	Natural antispasmodic effects on GI smooth muscles.	Alleviation of abdominal pain, bloating, and spasms in IBS.	Heartburn, potential allergic reactions.

DRUGS AFFECTING THE BILIARY SYSTEM:-

The biliary system, also known as the biliary tract, is a network of interconnected organs and ducts that play a vital role in the digestion and metabolism of fats in the body. It is responsible for the production, storage, and transportation of bile, a fluid essential for the digestion and absorption of dietary fats and fat-soluble vitamins (A, D, E, and K). The primary components of the biliary system include the liver, gallbladder, bile ducts, and sphincter of Oddi.

VOMITING:-

The act of vomiting is a physical event that results in the forceful **evacuation of gastric contents through the mouth**. It is often preceded by nausea (a feeling of 'queaziness' or of impending vomiting) and can be accompanied by retching (repetitive contraction of the abdominal muscles with or without actual discharge of vomit).

Vomiting can be a valuable (indeed life-saving) physiological response to the ingestion of a toxic substance (e.g. alcohol), but it is also an unwanted side-effect of many clinically used drugs, notably in patients receiving cancer chemotherapy.

Vomiting also occurs in early pregnancy, in the form of motion sickness and accompanies numerous disease states (e.g. migraine) and also bacterial and viral infections.

THE REFLEX MECHANISM OF VOMITING

Vomiting, also known as emesis is a complex reflex mechanism involving several organs and systems in the body. The primary purpose of vomiting is to expel harmful or irritating substances from the stomach and upper gastrointestinal tract. The reflex mechanism of vomiting is orchestrated by the brain and coordinated by the vomiting center, which is located in the medulla oblongata of the brainstem. Here is an overview of the reflex mechanism of vomiting:

1. Triggering Factors: Vomiting can be initiated by various triggers, including:
   - Stimulation of the chemoreceptor trigger zone (CTZ) in the brain by toxins, medications, or substances that can irritate the stomach lining.
   - Irritation of the stomach or upper gastrointestinal tract due to infections, inflammation, or mechanical obstruction.
2. Psychological factors, such as strong emotions or anxiety.
3. Receptor Activation: Receptors in the gastrointestinal tract and elsewhere in the body detect these triggers and send signals to the vomiting center. Some of these receptors include stretch receptors in the stomach, chemoreceptors in the CTZ, and sensory receptors in the throat.
4. Vomiting Center Activation: The vomiting center in the medulla oblongata receives input from these receptors and initiates the vomiting reflex. It coordinates the series of events that lead to vomiting.
5. Anti-Peristalsis: The vomiting center sends signals to the gastrointestinal muscles to initiate anti-peristalsis, which is the reverse of the normal peristaltic wave that pushes food downward. This action helps to move the stomach contents in the opposite direction, back up into the esophagus.
6. Closure of the Glottis: The glottis, a part of the larynx that controls the flow of air into the windpipe (trachea), closes to prevent the entry of vomit into the respiratory system. This is an important protective mechanism to avoid aspiration (inhaling vomit).
7. Retroperistalsis: The abdominal muscles contract forcefully, squeezing the stomach contents upward. This, combined with the anti-peristalsis, pushes the contents from the stomach into the esophagus.
8. Opening of the Lower Esophageal Sphincter (LES): The LES, which normally prevents the backflow of stomach contents into the esophagus, relaxes to allow the vomit to enter the esophagus.
9. Ejection of Vomit: The contents of the stomach are forcefully expelled from the mouth through the opened mouth and relaxed upper esophageal sphincter (UES).

10. Relief and Recovery: After vomiting, the individual typically experiences relief from the nausea or irritants that triggered the reflex. The body's goal is to remove the offending substances.

11. Potential Effects: Vomiting can be accompanied by various effects, including salivation, sweating, and increased heart rate. It can also cause a variety of sensations and discomfort.

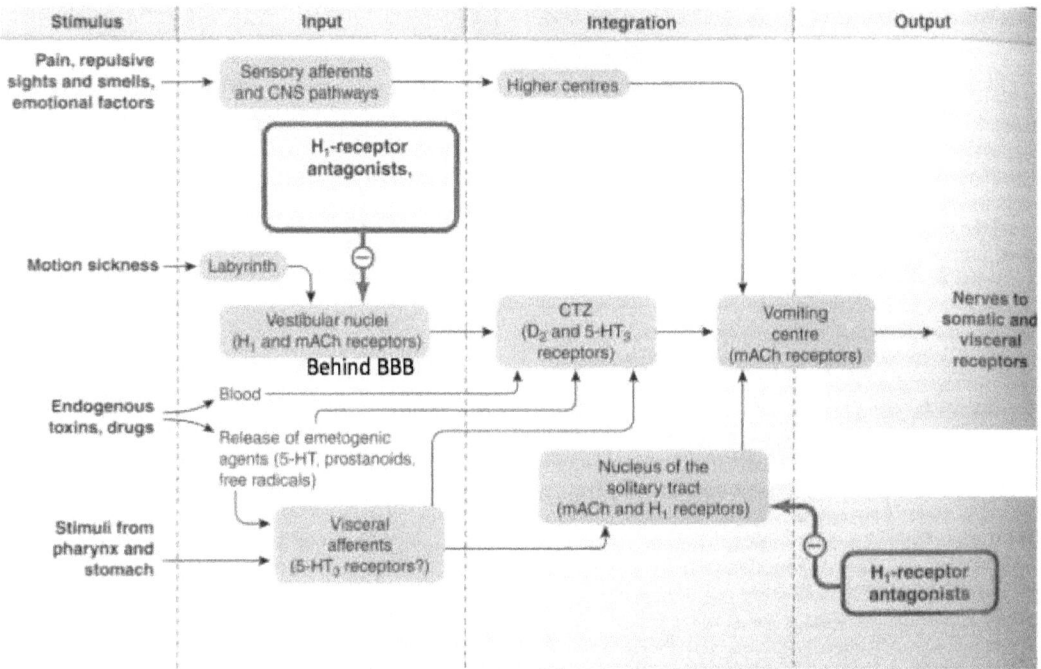

Fig. 8 THE REFLEX MECHANISM OF VOMITING

1. Laxatives /Purgatives

- A laxative is a medicine that loosens the bowel contents and encourages evacuation of stool.

- Laxatives / aperients are agents having milder action and helps in elimination of soft but formed stools. Purgatives / cathartics are agents having stronger action resulting in more fluid evacuation.

- Veterinarians use laxatives to help animals evacuate stool without excessive straining, to treat chronic constipation from nondietary causes and movable intestinal blockages (such as hair balls), and to evacuate the GI tract before surgery, radiography, or proctoscopy.

Below is a table 7 classifying laxatives or purgatives based on their main mechanisms of action:

Mechanism of Action	Example Laxatives/Purgatives
Bulk-forming agents	Psyllium, Methylcellulose
Osmotic laxatives	Polyethylene glycol (PEG), Magnesium citrate, Sorbitol, Lactulose
Stimulant laxatives	Bisacodyl, Senna, Cascara sagrada
Stool softeners	Docusate sodium
Lubricant laxatives	Mineral oil
Saline laxatives	Magnesium hydroxide (Milk of Magnesia)
Chloride channel activators	Lubiprostone
Guanylate cyclase-C agonists	Linaclotide

Bulk Forming

Bulk-forming laxatives are a type of medication or dietary supplement that is used to treat constipation and promote regular bowel movements. They work by increasing the bulk or volume of stool, which softens and expands the stool, making it easier to pass. These laxatives are generally considered safe and are often recommended for individuals with mild to moderate constipation. Here's how bulk-forming laxatives work and some examples:

Mechanism of Action:

Bulk-forming laxatives contain soluble fiber that is not digested in the small intestine. Instead, they absorb water in the colon, forming a soft and bulky stool. This increased stool volume stimulates the bowel to move and helps alleviate constipation. By promoting regular bowel movements, bulk-forming laxatives can also be useful in managing certain digestive disorders, such as irritable bowel syndrome (IBS) and diverticulosis.

Examples of Bulk-Forming Laxatives:

Psyllium (Metamucil): Psyllium is a natural fiber derived from the husks of psyllium seeds. It's available in various forms, including powder and capsules. When mixed with water, psyllium forms a gel-like substance that adds bulk to the stool.

Methylcellulose (Citrucel): Methylcellulose is another soluble fiber that, when ingested with water, swells in the intestines, aiding in the passage of stool.

Polycarbophil (FiberCon): Polycarbophil is another synthetic fiber that works similarly to psyllium and methylcellulose.

Indications:

Bulk-forming laxatives are primarily used to treat and prevent constipation. They are also recommended for individuals who need to soften their stool for medical reasons, such as after surgery or childbirth. These laxatives can help with the management of conditions like IBS and diverticulosis.

Adverse Effects:

Bulk-forming laxatives are generally well-tolerated, but some individuals may experience side effects, such as bloating, flatulence, and abdominal discomfort. It's important to take them with sufficient water to prevent them from causing an obstruction in the esophagus or intestines. If overused, they may lead to diarrhea or dehydration.

Osmotic (or hyperosmolar)

Osmotic laxatives, also known as hyperosmotic laxatives, are a type of medication used to relieve constipation. They work by drawing water into the colon or intestines, softening the stool and increasing the volume of intestinal contents. This promotes bowel movements by stimulating peristalsis and easing the passage of stool. Osmotic laxatives are generally effective for individuals with mild to moderate constipation. Here's how they work and some common examples:

Mechanism of Action:

Osmotic laxatives function by creating an osmotic gradient within the gastrointestinal tract. They contain substances that are not absorbed by the body, such as various salts or sugars, which retain water in the intestine. This additional water in the gut softens the stool, increases its volume, and triggers peristalsis, ultimately promoting bowel movements.

Examples of Osmotic Laxatives:

Magnesium Hydroxide (Milk of Magnesia): This medication contains magnesium ions that draw water into the intestines, leading to bowel movements. It is available as a liquid suspension.

Magnesium Citrate: Similar to milk of magnesia, magnesium citrate contains magnesium ions and is available as an oral solution. It's often used for bowel preparation before medical procedures or surgeries.

Sorbitol and Mannitol: These sugar alcohols have osmotic properties and are available as oral solutions or chewable tablets.

Lactulose: Lactulose is a synthetic sugar that is not absorbed by the small intestine. It is often prescribed to treat constipation and hepatic encephalopathy.

Polyethylene Glycol (MiraLAX): Polyethylene glycol is a tasteless, odorless powder that dissolves in water. It is used to relieve constipation and is available over the counter.

Indications:

Osmotic laxatives are primarily used to treat and prevent constipation. They are also sometimes used in medical settings for bowel cleansing before diagnostic tests, surgery, or colonoscopy.

Stimulant

Stimulant (irritant or contact) laxatives increase peristalsis by chemically irritating sensory nerve endings in the intestinal mucosa.

Bisacodyl (Dulcolax®), a cathartic that comes in enteric-coated and suppository forms. Castor oil (active ingredient: ricinoleic acid).

Ricinoleic acid inhibits water and electrolyte absorption, leading to fluid accumulation in the gastrointestinal tract and increased peristalsis.

Protectants/Adsorbents

This category of antidiarrheal drugs works either by coating inflamed intestinal mucosa with a protective layer (protectants), or by binding bacteria and/or digestive enzymes and/or toxins to protect intestinal mucosa from their damaging effects (adsorbents bind substances

Opiate or Narcotic Analgesic

Opiates or narcotic analgesics control diarrhea by decreasing both intestinal secretions and the flow of feces, and increasing segmental contractions, thereby resulting in increased intestinal absorption.

Side effects of these drugs include CNS depression (excitement in horses and cats), ileus, urinary retention, bloat, and constipation with prolonged use.

Probiotics

- Lactobacillus spp., Enterococcus faecium, and Bifidobacterium spp.
- The mechanisms of action of probiotics may involve competing with pathogenic bacteria for colonizing sites, production of antimicrobial factors, alteration of the microenvironment, reduction of local inflammation, and alteration of immune responses.
- Plain yogurt, Fastrack® gel, FortiFlora®, ProviableTM-DC, dsb.

Antifoaming / Antiflatulent Agents

Antifoaming or antiflatulent agents are substances used to reduce or prevent excessive gas or foam in the digestive system, which can lead to symptoms such as bloating, discomfort, and flatulence (passing gas). These agents help to break down or eliminate gas bubbles in the gastrointestinal tract, providing relief from gas-related symptoms. Here are some common antifoaming agents:

Simethicone:

Mechanism of Action: Simethicone is an over-the-counter antiflatulent that works by altering the surface tension of gas bubbles in the stomach and intestines. This causes the gas bubbles to combine and form larger, more easily eliminated gas bubbles, allowing for their expulsion and reducing the sensation of bloating and discomfort.

Indications: It is used to relieve gas-related symptoms, including bloating, abdominal discomfort, and excessive flatulence.

Adverse Effects: Simethicone is generally well-tolerated and has minimal side effects. It is considered safe for most individuals.

Activated Charcoal:

Mechanism of Action: Activated charcoal is sometimes used as an antiflatulent due to its ability to adsorb gas and gas-producing substances in the digestive system. It can help reduce gas-related symptoms.

Indications: Activated charcoal is less commonly used than simethicone and is typically used for specific cases of excessive gas or flatulence.

Adverse Effects: Possible side effects of activated charcoal can include constipation and black stools. It may interfere with the absorption of certain medications and should be used with caution.

Digestive Enzymes:

Mechanism of Action: Certain digestive enzyme supplements, such as alpha-galactosidase (found in products like Beano), help break down complex carbohydrates, such as those in beans and cruciferous vegetables, which can be a source of gas production.

Indications: Digestive enzyme supplements may be used to reduce gas and bloating associated with specific foods.

Adverse Effects: These supplements are typically well-tolerated, but they may not be effective for all types of gas.

DRUGS ACTING ON CNS

Agents used in the treatment of Parkinsonian disorders the classification of these drugs includes:

The treatment of Parkinsonian disorders, such as Parkinson's disease, involves a variety of medications that aim to alleviate the motor symptoms and improve the quality of life for individuals affected by these conditions. These medications can be classified into several categories based on their mechanisms of action. Here is a classification of drugs used in the treatment of Parkinsonian disorders:

Dopaminergic Agents:

Dopamine Precursors: These drugs are converted into dopamine in the brain, helping to replenish the depleted dopamine levels in Parkinson's disease.

Levodopa (L-DOPA) is the primary example.

Dopamine Agonists: These medications mimic the effects of dopamine in the brain, stimulating dopamine receptors.

Examples include pramipexole, ropinirole, and apomorphine.

MAO-B Inhibitors (Monoamine Oxidase B Inhibitors):

These drugs inhibit the enzyme monoamine oxidase B, which breaks down dopamine in the brain, thus increasing dopamine levels.

Examples include selegiline and rasagiline.

COMT Inhibitors (Catechol-O-Methyltransferase Inhibitors):

These drugs block the action of the enzyme catechol-O-methyltransferase, which metabolizes levodopa, allowing more levodopa to reach the brain.

Entacapone and tolcapone are examples.

Anticholinergic Agents:

These drugs reduce the activity of acetylcholine, a neurotransmitter that becomes imbalanced in Parkinson's disease.

Examples include trihexyphenidyl and benztropine.

Amantadine:

Amantadine is an antiviral medication that also has dopaminergic effects and can help manage symptoms in Parkinson's disease.

Antiviral Drugs:

In some cases, antiviral drugs may be used to treat specific parkinsonian disorders, such as parkinsonism induced by certain viral infections.

Non-Dopaminergic Agents:

These drugs do not directly affect dopamine levels but may be used to address certain non-motor symptoms or as adjunctive therapy.

Examples include clozapine for psychosis and medications to address mood and sleep disturbances.

Surgical Interventions:

In advanced cases of Parkinson's disease, surgical options such as deep brain stimulation (DBS) may be considered. DBS involves implanting electrodes in specific brain regions to modulate abnormal neural activity.

Below is a table 8 listing some of the common agents used in the treatment of Parkinson's disease and other Parkinsonian disorders:

Class of Medication	Examples of Medications
Dopamine Precursors	Levodopa (L-dopa)
Dopamine Agonists	Pramipexole, Ropinirole, Apomorphine
MAO-B Inhibitors	Rasagiline, Selegiline
COMT Inhibitors	Entacapone, Tolcapone
Anticholinergics	Trihexyphenidyl, Benztropine
Amantadine	Amantadine
NMDA Receptor Antagonist	Amantadine (also acts on NMDA receptors)

It's important to note that the choice of medication and treatment approach for Parkinson's disease and other Parkinsonian disorders depends on various factors, including the patient's age, overall health, disease severity, and the presence of other medical conditions. Treatment plans are often individualized and may involve combinations of different medications to address the specific symptoms and needs of the patient. The use of these medications should be carefully managed by a neurologist or movement disorder specialist experienced in Parkinson's disease management.

ANTI VIRAL DRUG CLASSIFICATION

The replication of viruses depends on synthetic processes of the host cell. Antiviral drugs can exert their actions at several stages of viral replication including viral entry, nucleic acid synthesis and integration, late protein synthesis, and processing, as well as in the final stages of viral packaging and virion release (Figure 49–1). Most of the drugs active against herpes viruses (HSV) and many agents active against human immunodeficiency virus (HIV) are antimetabolites, structurally similar to naturally occurring compounds. The selective toxicity of antiviral drugs usually depends on greater susceptibility of viral enzymes to their inhibitory actions than host cell enzymes.

One of the most important trends in viral chemotherapy, especially in the management of HIV infection, has been the introduction of combination drug therapy. This can result in greater clinical effectiveness in viral infections and can also prevent, or delay, the emergence of resistance.

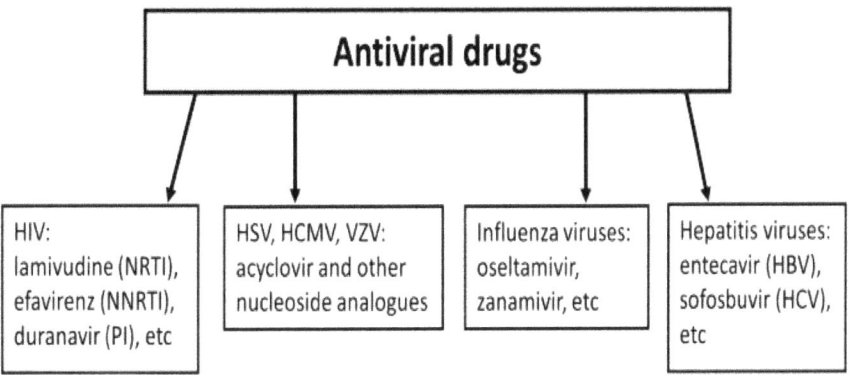

ANTIHERPES DRUGS

Most drugs active against herpes viruses are antimetabolites bioactivated via viral or host cell kinases to form compounds that inhibit viral DNA polymerases.

A. Acyclovir (Acycloguanosine)

1. Mechanisms

Acyclovir is a guanosine analog active against herpes simplex virus (HSV1, HSV2) and varicellazoster virus (VZV). The drug is activated initially by the viral kinase to form acyclovir triphosphate, which interferes with viral synthesis in 2 ways. It acts as a competitive substrate for DNA polymerase, and it leads to chain termination after its incorporation into viral DNA (Figure 49–2). Resistance of HSV can involve changes in viral DNA polymerase. However, many resistant strains of HSV (TK–strains) lack thymidine kinase, the enzyme involved in the initial viralspecific phosphorylation of acyclovir. Such strains are crossresistant to famciclovir, ganciclovir, and valacyclovir.

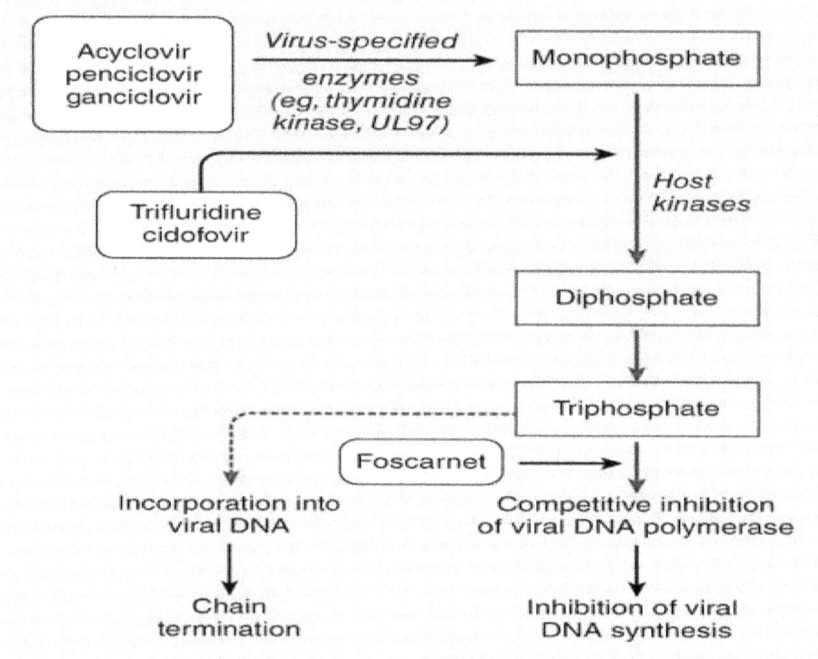

Fig. 9 Illustrations of Acyclovir Mechanism

2. Pharmacokinetics

Acyclovir can be administered by the topical, oral, and intravenous routes. Because of its short halflife, oral administration requires multiple daily doses of acyclovir.

Renal excretion is the major route of elimination of acyclovir, and dosage should be reduced in patients with renal impairment.

3. **Clinical uses and toxicity**

Oral acyclovir is commonly used for the treatment of mucocutaneous and genital herpes lesions (Table 49–1) and for prophylaxis in AIDS and in other immunocompromised patients (eg, those undergoing organ transplantation). The oral drug is well tolerated but may cause gastrointestinal (GI) distress and headache. Intravenous administration is used for severe herpes disease, including encephalitis, and for neonatal HSV infection. Toxic effects with parenteral administration include delirium, tremor, seizures, hypotension, and nephrotoxicity. Acyclovir has no significant toxicity on the bone marrow. Table 8

Virus	Primary Drugs	Alternative or Adjunctive Drugs
CMV	Ganciclovir, valganciclovir	Cidofovir, foscarnet, fomivirsen
HSV, VZV	Acyclovira	Cidofovir, foscarnet, vidarabine
HBV	IFNα, lamivudine	Adefovir dipivoxil, entecavir, lamivudine, telbivudine
HCV	IFNα, sofosbuvir	Ledipasvir, grazoprevir, ribavirin
Influenza A	Oseltamivir	Amantadine, rimantadine, zanamivir
Influenza B	Oseltamivir	Zanamivir

aAntiHSV drugs similar to acyclovir include famciclovir, penciclovir, and valacyclovir; IFNα, interferonα.

4. **Other drugs for HSV and VSV infections**

Several newer agents have characteristics similar to those of acyclovir. Valacyclovir is a prodrug converted to acyclovir by hepatic metabolism after oral administration and reaches plasma levels 3–5 times greater than those achieved by acyclovir. Valacyclovir has a longer duration of action than acyclovir. Penciclovir undergoes activation by viral thymidine kinase, and the triphosphate form inhibits DNA polymerase but does not cause chain termination. Famciclovir is a prodrug converted to penciclovir by firstpass metabolism in the liver. Used orally in genital herpes and for herpes zoster, famciclovir is well tolerated and is similar to acyclovir in its pharmacokinetic properties. None of the acyclovir congeners has activity against TK– strains of HSV. Docosanol is an aliphatic alcohol that inhibits fusion between the HSV envelope and plasma membranes. It prevents viral entry and subsequent replication. Used topically, docosanol shortens healing time.

B. Ganciclovir

1. Mechanisms

Ganciclovir, a guanine derivative, is triphosphorylated to form a nucleotide that inhibits DNA polymerases of cytomegalovirus (CMV) and HSV and causes chain termination. The first phosphorylation step is catalyzed by virusspecific enzymes in both CMV infected and HSVinfected cells. CMV resistance mechanisms involve mutations in the genes that code for the activating viral phosphotransferase and the viral DNA polymerase. Thymidine kinase deficient HSV strains are resistant to ganciclovir.

2. Pharmacokinetics

Ganciclovir is usually given intravenously and penetrates well into tissues, including the eye and the central nervous system (CNS). The drug undergoes renal elimination in direct proportion to creatinine clearance. Oral bioavailability is less than 10%. An intraocular implant form of ganciclovir can be used in CMV retinitis. Valganciclovir, a prodrug of ganciclovir, has high oral bioavailability and has decreased the use of intravenous forms of ganciclovir (and also of intravenous cidofovir and foscarnet) in endorgan CMV disease.

3. Clinical uses and toxicity

Ganciclovir is used for the prophylaxis and treatment of CMV retinitis and other CMV infections in immunocompromised patients. Systemic toxic effects include leukopenia, thrombocytopenia, mucositis, hepatic dysfunction, and seizures. The drug may cause severe neutropenia when used with

E. Other Antiherpes Drugs

1. Vidarabine

Vidarabine is an adenine analog and has activity against HSV, VZV, and CMV. Its use for systemic infections is limited by rapid metabolic inactivation and marked toxic potential. Vidarabine is used topically for herpes keratitis but has no effect on genital lesions. Toxic effects with systemic use include GI irritation, paresthesias, tremor, convulsions, and hepatic dysfunction. Vidarabine is teratogenic in animals.

2. Idoxuridine and trifluridine

These pyrimidine analogs are used topically in herpes keratitis (HSV1). They are too toxic for systemic use.

3. Fomivirsen

Fomivirsen is an antisense oligonucleotide that binds to mRNA of CMV, inhibiting early protein synthesis. The drug is injected intravitreally for treatment of CMV retinitis rossresistance between fomivirsen and other antiCMV agents has not been observed. Concurrent systemic antiCMV therapy is recommended to protect against extraocular and contralateral retinal CMV disease. Fomivirsen causes iritis, vitreitis, increased intraocular pressure and changes in vision.

Here is a list of common antiviral drugs used to treat herpes infections in a table 9:

Drug Name	Brand Names	Type of Herpes Infection Treated
Acyclovir	Zovirax	Herpes simplex virus (HSV)
Valacyclovir	Valtrex	HSV, herpes zoster (shingles)
Famciclovir	Famvir	HSV, herpes zoster (shingles)
Penciclovir	Denavir	HSV (topical treatment for cold sores)
Docosanol	Abreva	HSV (topical treatment for cold sores)
Ganciclovir	Cytovene, Zirgan	Cytomegalovirus (CMV) in immunocompromised individuals
Foscarnet	Foscavir	CMV, HSV, varicella-zoster virus (VZV)

Valganciclovir	Valcyte	CMV (used when oral therapy is preferred)
Brincidofovir	Brincidofovir	CMV and other DNA viruses in immunocompromised individuals
Letermovir	Prevymis	CMV prophylaxis in hematopoietic stem cell transplant patients

These antiviral drugs work by interfering with the replication and spread of the herpes simplex virus (HSV) and other related viruses, including varicella-zoster virus (VZV) and cytomegalovirus (CMV). Some of these medications are available in both oral and topical forms, and the choice of drug and route of administration depends on the specific condition being treated. It's important to use these medications as prescribed by a healthcare professional, as they can help manage symptoms and reduce the frequency and severity of herpes outbreaks.

ANTI-HIV DRUGS

The main drugs effective against HIV are antimetabolite inhibitors of viral reverse transcriptase and inhibitors of viral aspartate protease.

The current approach to treating HIV infection involves initiating treatment with three or more antiretroviral drugs, if possible, before symptoms appear. These drug combinations typically include nucleoside reverse transcriptase inhibitors (NRTIs) along with HIV protease inhibitors (PIs). This therapeutic strategy is known as Highly Active Antiretroviral Therapy (HAART).

HAART, involving drug combinations, aims to slow or reverse the increase in viral RNA load typically observed during the progression of the disease. It also helps to slow or reverse the decline in CD4 cells and reduces the incidence of opportunistic infections in many AIDS patients.

The combination of multiple antiretroviral drugs helps to suppress viral replication effectively and reduce the viral load in the body. This approach is critical in managing HIV infection and improving the quality of life for individuals living with HIV. By targeting different stages of the viral life cycle, HAART has been instrumental in extending the life expectancy and reducing the mortality associated with HIV/AIDS. TABLE 10

Subclasses	Prototype	Other significant Agents
Nucleoside reverse transcriptase inhibitors	zidovudine	Abacavir, didanosine, emtricitabine, lamivudine, stavudine, zalcitabine
Nonnucleoside reverse transcriptase inhibitors	Delvirdine	Efavirenz, etravirine, nevirapine, rilpivirine, tenofovir

Protease inhibitors	Indinavir	Amprenavir, atazanavir, darunavir, lopinavir, nelfinavir, ritonavir, saquinavir, tipranavir
CCR5 antagonist	Mariviroc	
Fusion inhibitor	Enfervutide	

A. Nucleoside Reverse Transcriptase Inhibitors (NRTIs)

To convert their RNA into dsDNA, retroviruses require virally encoded RNAdependent DNA polymerase (reverse transcriptase). Mammalian RNA and DNA polymerases are sufficiently distinct to permit a selective inhibition of the viral reverse transcriptase.

NRTIs are prodrugs converted by host cell kinases to triphosphates, which not only competitively inhibit binding of natural nucleotides to the Deoxyribonucleotide triphosphate (dNTP)binding site of reverse transcriptase but also act as chain terminators via their insertion into the growing DNA chain. Because NRTIs lack a 3′hydroxyl

Group on the ribose ring, attachment of the next nucleotide is impossible. Resistance emerges rapidly when NRTIs are used as single agents via mutations in the pol gene; crossresistance occurs but is not complete.

1. Abacavir

A guanosine analog, abacavir has good oral bioavailability and an intracellular halflife of 12–24 h. HIV resistance requires several concomitant mutations and tends to develop slowly. Hypersensitivity reactions, occasionally fatal, occur in 5% of HIV patients.

2. Didanosine (ddI)

Oral bioavailability of ddI is reduced by food and by chelating agents. The drug is eliminated by the kidney, and the dose must be reduced in patients with renal dysfunction. Pancreatitis is dose limiting and occurs more frequently in alcoholic patients and those with hypertriglyceridemia. Other adverse effects include peripheral neuropathy, diarrhea, hepatic dysfunction, hyperuricemia, and CNS effects.

3. Emtricitabine

Good oral bioavailability and renal elimination with long halflife permit oncedaily dosing of emtricitabine. Because of the propylene glycol in the oral solution, the drug is contraindicated in pregnancy and young children and in patients with hepatic or renal dysfunction. Common adverse effects of the drug include asthenia, GI distress, headache, and hyperpigmentation of the palms and/or the soles.

4. Lamivudine (3T C)

Lamivudine is 80% bioavailable by the oral route and is eliminated almost exclusively by the kidney. In addition to its use in HAART regimens for HIV, lamivudine is also effective in hepatitis B infections. Dosage adjustment is needed in patients with renal insufficiency. **Adverse effects of lamivudine** are usually mild and include GI distress, headache, insomnia, and fatigue.

Stavudine has good oral bioavailability and penetrates most tissues, including the CNS. Dosage adjustment is needed in renal insufficiency. Peripheral neuropathy is doselimiting and increased with coadministration of didanosine or zalcitabine. Lactic acidosis with hepatic steatosis occurs more frequently with stavudine than with other NRTIs.

6. Tenofovir

Although it is a nucleotide, tenofovir acts like NRTIs to competitively inhibit reverse transcriptase and cause chain termination after incorporation into DNA. Tenofovir also has activity against HBV (see below). Oral bioavailability of tenofovir is in the 25–40% range, the intracellular halflife is more than 60 h, and the drug undergoes renal elimination. Tenofovir may impede the renal elimination of acyclovir and ganciclovir. Adverse effects include GI distress, asthenia, and headache; rare cases of acute renal failure and Fanconi's syndrome have been reported.

7. Zalcitabine (ddC)

Zalcitabine has a high oral bioavailability. Dosage adjustment is needed in patients with renal insufficiency and nephrotoxic drugs (eg, amphotericin B, aminoglycosides) increase toxic potential. Doselimiting peripheral neuropathy is the major adverse effect of ddC. Pancreatitis, esophageal ulceration, stomatitis, and arthralgias may also occur.

8. Zidovudine (Z D V)

Formerly called azidothymidine (AZT), zidovudine is active orally and is distributed to most tissues, including the CNS. Elimination of the drug involves both hepatic metabolism to glucuronides and renal excretion. Dosage reduction is necessary in uremic patients and those with cirrhosis. The primary toxicity of zidovudine is bone marrow suppression (additive with other immunosuppressive drugs) leading to anemia and neutropenia, which may require transfusions. GI distress, thrombocytopenia, headaches, myalgia, acute cholestatic hepatitis, agitation, and insomnia may also occur. Drugs that may increase plasma levels of zidovudine include azole antifungals and protease inhibitors. Rifampin increases the clearance of zidovudine.

9. NRTIs and lactic acidosis

NRTI agents, taken alone or in combination with other antiretroviral agents, may cause lactic acidemia and severe hepatomegaly with steatosis. Risk factors include obesity, prolonged treatment with NRTIs, and preexisting liver dysfunction. Consideration should be given to suspension of NRTI treatment in patients who develop elevated aminotransferase levels.

B. Nonnucleoside Reverse Transcriptase Inhibitors (NNRTIs)

NNRTIs bind to a site on reverse transcriptase different from the binding site of NRTIs. Nonnucleoside drugs do not require phosphorylation to be active and do not compete with nucleoside triphosphates. There is no crossresistance with NRTIs. Resistance from mutations in the pol gene occurs very rapidly if these agents are used as monotherapy.

1. Delavirdine

Drug interactions are a major problem with delavirdine, which is metabolized by both CYP3A4 and CYP2D6. Its blood levels are decreased by antacids, ddI, phenytoin, rifampin, and nelfinavir. Conversely, the blood levels of delavirdine are increased by azole antifungals and macrolide antibiotics. Delavirdine increases plasma levels of several benzodiazepines, nifedipine, protease inhibitors, quinidine, and warfarin. Delavirdine causes skin rash in up to 20% of patients, and the drug should be avoided in pregnancy because it is teratogenic in animals.

2. Efavirenz

Efavirenz can be given once daily because of its long halflife. Fatty foods may enhance its oral bioavailability. Efavirenz is metabolized by hepatic cytochromes P450 and is frequently involved in drug interactions. Toxicity of efavirenz includes CNS dysfunction, skin rash, and elevations of plasma cholesterol. Efavirenz is one of the NNRTI agents recommended for use in pregnancy, but should be initiated after the first 8 weeks due to birth defects observed in a primate study at doses similar to those used in humans.

3. Etravirine

Etravirine is approved for treatmentexperienced HIV patients, and may be effective against HIV strains resistant to other drugs in the group. The drug causes rash, nausea, and diarrhea. Elevations in serum cholesterol, triglycerides, and transaminase levels may occur. Etravirine is a substrate as well as an inducer of CYP3A4 and also inhibits CYP2C9 and CYP2C19 and may be involved in significant drug drug interactions.

4. Nevirapine

Nevirapine has good oral bioavailability, penetrates most tissues including the CNS, has a halflife of more than 24 h, and is metabolized by the hepatic CYP3A4 isoform. The drug is used in combination regimens and is effective in preventing HIV vertical transmission when given as single doses to mothers at the onset of labor and to the neonate. Hypersensitivity reactions with nevirapine include a rash, which occurs in 15–20% of patients, especially females. StevensJohnson syndrome and a lifethreatening toxic epidermal necrolysis have also been reported. Nevirapine blood levels are increased by cimetidine and macrolide antibiotics and decreased by enzyme inducers such as rifampin.

5. Rilpivirine

Rilpivirine is a highly proteinbound diarylpyrimidine with a long halflife of 50 h. Its oral bioavailability is dependent on an acid gastric environment for optimal absorption; thus antacids and H2receptor antagonists should be separated in time and proton pump inhibitors are contraindicated. Rilpivirine is one of the NNRTI agents recommended for use in pregnancy. Rilpivirine is primarily metabolized by CYP3A4, and drugs that induce or inhibit CYP3A4 may thus affect the clearance of rilpivirine. The most common adverse effects associated with rilpivirine therapy are rash, depression, headache, insomnia, and increased serum aminotransferases. Increased serum cholesterol and fat redistribution syndrome have also been reported. Higher doses have been associated with QTc prolongation.

C. Protease Inhibitors

The assembly of infectious HIV virions is dependent on an aspartate protease (HIV1 protease) encoded by the pol gene. This viral enzyme cleaves precursor polyproteins to form the final structural proteins of the mature virion core. The HIV protease inhibitors are designer drugs based on molecular characterization of the active site of the viral enzyme. Resistance is mediated via multiple point mutations in the pol gene; the extent of crossresistance is variable depending on the specific protease inhibitor. Protease inhibitors (PIs) have important clinical use in AIDS, most commonly in combinations with reverse transcriptase inhibitors as components of HAART. All of the PIs are substrates and inhibitors of CYP3A4 with ritonavir having the most pronounced inhibitory effect. The PIs are implicated in many drugdrug interactions with other antiretroviral agents and with commonly used medications.

1. Atazanavir

This is a PI with a pharmacokinetic profile that permits oncedaily dosing. Oral absorption of atazanavir requires an acidic environment—antacid ingestion should be separated by 12 h. The drug penetrates cerebrospinal and seminal fluids and undergoes biliary elimination. **Adverse effects** include GI distress, peripheral neuropathy, skin rash, and hyperbilirubinemia. Prolongation of the QTc interval may occur at high doses. Unlike most PIs, atazanavir does not appear to be associated with dyslipidemias, fat deposition, or a metabolic syndrome. However, it is a potent inhibitor of **CYP3A4, CYP2C9, and UGT1A1**.

2. Darunavir

This drug is used in combination with ritonavir or cobicistat in treatmentexperienced patients with resistance to other PIs. The drug is a substrate of CYP3A4. GI adverse effects and rash occur, and liver toxicity has been reported. Darunavir contains a sulfonamide moiety and should be used with caution in patients with sulfonamide allergy.

3. Fosamprenavir

Fosamprenavir is a prodrug, forming amprenavir via its hydrolysis in the GI tract. The drug formulation includes propylene glycol and should not be used in children or in pregnant women. Fosamprenavir is often used in combination with lowdose ritonavir. The absorption of amprenavir is impeded by fatty foods. Amprenavir undergoes hepatic metabolism and is both an inhibitor and an inducer of CYP3A4. The drug causes GI distress, paresthesias, and rash, the latter sometimes severe enough to warrant drug discontinuation. Cross allergenicity may occur with sulfonamides.

4. Indinavir

Oral bioavailability of indinavir is good except in the presence of food. Clearance is mainly via the liver, with about 10% renal excretion. Adverse effects include nausea, diarrhea, thrombocytopenia, hyperbilirubinemia, and nephrolithiasis. To reduce renal damage, it is important to maintain good hydration. Insulin resistance may be more common with indinavir than other PIs. Indinavir is a substrate for and an inhibitor of the cytochrome P450 isoform CYP3A4 and is implicated in drug interactions. Serum levels of indinavir are increased by azole antifungals and decreased by rifamycins. Indinavir increases the serum levels of antihistamines, benzodiazepines, and rifampin.

5. **Lopinavir/ritonavir** In this combination, a subtherapeutic dose of ritonavir acts as a pharmacokinetic enhancer ("booster") by inhibiting the CYP3A4mediated Metabolism of lopinavir. Patient compliance is improved owing to lower pill burden and the combination is usually well tolerated.

6. Nelfinavir

This PI is characterized by increased oral absorption in the presence of food, hepatic metabolism via CYP3A4, and a short halflife. As an inhibitor of drug metabolism, nelfinavir has been involved in many drug interactions. Adverse effects include diarrhea, which can be doselimiting. The drug has the most favorable safety profile of the PIs in pregnancy.

7. Ritonavir

Oral bioavailability is good, and the drug should be taken with meals. Clearance is mainly via the liver, and dosage reduction is necessary in patients with hepatic impairment. The most common adverse effects of ritonavir are GI irritation and a bitter taste. Paresthesias and elevations of hepatic aminotransferases and triglycerides in the plasma also occur. Drugs that increase the activity of the cytochrome P450 isoform CYP3A4 (anticonvulsants, rifamycins) reduce serum levels of ritonavir, and drugs that inhibit this enzyme (azole antifungals, cimetidine, erythromycin) elevate serum levels of the antiviral drug. Ritonavir inhibits the metabolism of a wide range of drugs, including erythromycin, dronabinol, ketoconazole, prednisone, rifampin, and saquinavir.Subtherapeutic doses of ritonavir inhibit the CYP3Amediated metabolism of other protease inhibitors (eg, indinavir, lopinavir, saquinavir); this is the rationale for PI combinations that include ritonavir because it permits the use of lower doses of the other protease inhibitor.

8. Saquinavir

Original formulations of saquinavir had low and erratic oral bioavailability. Reformulation for once daily dosing in combination with lowdose ritonavir has improved efficacy with decreased GI side effects. The drug undergoes extensive firstpass metabolism and functions as both a substrate and inhibitor of CYP3A4. Adverse effects of saquinavir include nausea, diarrhea, dyspepsia, and rhinitis. Saquinavir plasma levels are increased by azole antifungals, clarithromycin, grapefruit juice, indinavir, and ritonavir. Drugs that induce CYP3A4 decrease plasma levels of saquinavir.

9. Tipranavir

This is a newer drug used in combination with ritonavir in treatmentexperienced patients with resistance to other PIs. The drug is a substrate and inducer of CYP3A4 and also induces Pglycoprotein transporters, possibly altering GI absorption of other drugs. For example, increased blood levels of the HMGCoA reductase inhibitors (eg, lovastatin) may occur, thus increasing the risk for myopathy and rhabdomyolysis. GI adverse effects, rash, and liver toxicity have been reported.

10. Effects on carbohydrate and lipid metabolism

The use of PIs in HAART drug combinations has led to the development of disorders in carbohydrate and lipid metabolism. It has been suggested that this is due to the inhibition of lipidregulating proteins, which have active sites with structural homology to that of HIV protease. The syndrome includes hyperglycemia and insulin resistance or hyperlipidemia, with altered body fat distribution. Buffalo hump, gynecomastia, and truncal obesity may occur with facial and peripheral lipodystrophy. The syndrome has been observed with PIs used in HAART regimens, with an incidence of 30–50% and a median onset time of approximately 1 year duration of treatment. Atazanavir does not appear to be associated with dyslipidemia or hyperglycemia.

D. Entry and Fusion Inhibitors

1. Maraviroc HIV1 infection begins with attachment of an HIV envelope protein called gp120 to CD4 molecules on surfaces of helper T cells and other antigenpresenting cells such as macrophages and dendritic cells. The attachment of many HIV strains involves a transmembrane chemokine receptor CCR5 (ie, CCR5tropic HIV strains). This receptor, a human protein, is the target for maraviroc, which blocks viral attachment. Although resistance has occurred, there is minimal crossresistance with other antiretroviral drugs. Note that CXCR4tropic HIV is not affected by maraviroc so tropic testing of the virus is key. Maraviroc is used orally and has good tissue penetration. It is a substrate for CYP3A4, and dosage adjustments may be needed in the presence of drugs that induce or inhibit this enzyme. Adverse effects of maraviroc include cough, diarrhea, muscle and joint pain, and increases in hepatic transaminases.

2. Enfuvirtide

Enfuvirtide is a synthetic 36 aminoacid peptide. The drug binds to the gp41 subunit of the viral envelope glycoprotein, preventing the conformational changes required for the fusion of the viral and cellular membranes. There is no crossresistance with other antiHIV drugs, but resistance may occur via mutations in the env gene. Enfuvirtide is administered subcutaneously in combination with other antiHIV agents in previously drugtreated patients with persistent HIV1 replication despite ongoing therapy. Its metabolism via hydrolysis does not involve the cytochrome P450 system. injection site reactions and hypersensitivity may occur. An increased incidence of bacterial pneumonia has been reported.

E. Integrase Strand Transfer Inhibitors (INSTs) Raltegravir is a pyrimidine derivative that binds integrase, an enzyme essential to replication of both HIV1 and HIV2, inhibiting strand transfer. As a result, integration of reversetranscribed HIV DNA into host cell chromosomes is inhibited. The drug has been used mainly in treatmentnaïve HIV patients, usually in combination regimens. The drug is metabolized by glucuronidation and is not affected by agents that induce or inhibit hepatic cytochromes P450. However, if used with rifampin, which induces UDPglucuronosyltransferase, the dose of raltegravir should be doubled. Adverse effects include nausea, dizziness, and fatigue. An increase in creatinine kinase has been reported, with potential for myopathy or rhabdomyolysis. Dolutegravir and elvitegravir are similar.

ANTIINFLUENZA AGENTS

A. Amantadine and Rimantadine

Amantadine and rimantadine are antiviral medications primarily used for the prevention and treatment of influenza A virus infections. They belong to a class of drugs known as adamantane derivatives.

Mechanism of Action:

Amantadine and rimantadine work by interfering with the viral replication process of influenza A virus. They block a protein called the M2 ion channel in the viral envelope, which is essential for the release of viral genetic material (RNA) into the host cell during viral replication. By inhibiting the M2 ion channel, these drugs prevent the uncoating of the viral particles and the release of the viral genetic material, thereby inhibiting viral replication and spread.

Clinical Uses:

Influenza Prophylaxis: Amantadine and rimantadine are used for the prevention of influenza A virus infection in individuals who have not been vaccinated or are at high risk of influenza complications. However, their use for this purpose has become limited due to the emergence of viral resistance.

Influenza Treatment: These drugs are used for the treatment of uncomplicated influenza A virus infections in patients who have been symptomatic for no more than 48 hours. They can help reduce the duration and severity of flu symptoms when started early in the course of the illness.

It's important to note that amantadine and rimantadine are not effective against influenza B virus or other respiratory viruses. Additionally, the effectiveness of these drugs has decreased in recent years due to the emergence of resistant strains of influenza A virus. As a result, their use in the treatment of influenza is now more limited, and they are no longer recommended as first-line treatment options.

Safety Considerations:

Amantadine and rimantadine can have side effects, and their use should be monitored by a healthcare professional. Common side effects may include gastrointestinal upset, dizziness, and insomnia.

These drugs should be used with caution in individuals with certain medical conditions, such as epilepsy, glaucoma, or kidney disorders. They may also interact with other medications, and patients should inform their healthcare provider about all medications they are taking.

In recent years, due to the emergence of viral resistance and the availability of more effective antiviral drugs, such as neuraminidase inhibitors (oseltamivir and zanamivir), the use of amantadine and rimantadine has decreased in favor of other treatment options for influenza A. The choice of antiviral treatment for influenza should be guided by the latest clinical guidelines and the individual patient's condition.

B. Oseltamivir and Zanamivir

Oseltamivir and zanamivir are antiviral medications used for the treatment and prevention of influenza virus infections, specifically influenza A and influenza B. They belong to a class of drugs known as neuraminidase inhibitors.

Oseltamivir:

Mechanism of Action: Oseltamivir inhibits the neuraminidase enzyme on the surface of the influenza virus. Neuraminidase is essential for the release of new viral particles from infected cells. By blocking neuraminidase, oseltamivir prevents the spread of the virus to other cells in the body and reduces the severity and duration of influenza symptoms.

Clinical Uses:

Treatment of Influenza: Oseltamivir is used for the treatment of uncomplicated influenza in patients aged 2 weeks and older who have been symptomatic for no more than 48 hours.

Prophylaxis: It can be used as post-exposure prophylaxis to prevent influenza in individuals who have been in close contact with someone diagnosed with the flu.

Zanamivir:

Mechanism of Action: Zanamivir also inhibits the neuraminidase enzyme of the influenza virus, preventing viral release and spread within the body.

Clinical Uses:

Treatment of Influenza: Zanamivir is used for the treatment of uncomplicated influenza in patients aged 7 years and older who have been symptomatic for no more than 48 hours.

Prophylaxis: It can be used as post-exposure prophylaxis to prevent influenza in individuals who have been in close contact with someone diagnosed with the flu.

Route of Administration:

Oseltamivir: It is available as an oral capsule or suspension and is taken by mouth.

Zanamivir: It is available as an inhalation powder and is administered via oral inhalation using a special inhaler device.

Safety Considerations:

Oseltamivir and zanamivir are generally well-tolerated, but they may cause side effects such as nausea, vomiting, headache, and cough. Rarely, they may be associated with serious neuropsychiatric side effects in some individuals.

Individuals with asthma or chronic respiratory conditions should use zanamivir with caution due to the risk of bronchospasm.

Both oseltamivir and zanamivir are most effective when started early in the course of the illness, ideally within 48 hours of symptom onset. They are essential components of influenza management, particularly during seasonal outbreaks or in the context of a pandemic. However, it's important to note that antiviral treatment should be guided by healthcare professionals, and not all individuals with influenza require antiviral therapy.

Here is a list of common antiviral drugs used to treat and manage influenza (the flu) in a table 11:

Drug Name	Brand Names	Type of Influenza Virus Treated	Administration
Oseltamivir	Tamiflu	Influenza A and B	Oral
Zanamivir	Relenza	Influenza A and B	Inhaled
Peramivir	Rapivab	Influenza A and B	Intravenous
Baloxavir marboxil	Xofluza	Influenza A and B	Oral

These antiviral drugs are used to treat and manage influenza by inhibiting the replication of the influenza virus and reducing the severity and duration of symptoms. They are most effective when taken within the first 48 hours of symptom onset. The choice of drug and route of administration may depend on the specific circumstances and the patient's age and health status.

It's important to note that while antiviral drugs can help reduce the severity and duration of influenza symptoms, they are not a replacement for influenza vaccination, which is the most effective way to prevent the flu. Vaccination is recommended annually, especially for individuals at higher risk of complications from influenza.

AGENTS USED IN VIRAL HEPATITIS

The medications available for the treatment of infections caused by the hepatitis B virus (HBV) are suppressive in nature, meaning they aim to control the virus and prevent its replication, but they do not completely eliminate it from the body. On the other hand, drugs used for hepatitis C virus (HCV) infections have the primary goal of achieving viral eradication, which means completely eliminating the virus from the body.

A. IFNα

Mechanism

Interferon-alpha (IFNα) is a cytokine with antiviral properties used to treat viral infections like hepatitis B and hepatitis C. Its mechanisms of action include direct inhibition of viral replication, boosting the immune response against the virus, inducing cell death in infected cells, inhibiting viral entry, reducing inflammation, and promoting the production of host defense proteins. IFNα's diverse actions help control and clear viral infections, but it may have side effects and is often used in combination with other antiviral drugs for better treatment outcomes.

2. Pharmacokinetics

Interferon-alpha (IFNα) is a complex protein-based drug with unique pharmacokinetic characteristics IFNα can be administered via different routes, including subcutaneous injection, intramuscular injection, or intravenous infusion. The route of administration can influence the drug's absorption and distribution. Following subcutaneous or intramuscular injection, IFNα is slowly and gradually absorbed into the bloodstream. Intravenous administration results in immediate and complete drug availability in the systemic circulation IFNα is a large protein molecule, and it distributes extensively throughout the body after entering the bloodstream. It can penetrate various tissues and organs, including the liver, spleen, and bone marrow IFNα has a high affinity for binding to plasma proteins, which may affect its distribution and elimination from the body IFNα undergoes metabolism in various tissues, particularly in the liver and kidneys. However, the metabolism of IFNα is relatively limited compared to small-molecule drugs. IFNα is primarily eliminated from the body by renal clearance, which means it is filtered by the kidneys and excreted in the urine. Individual patient factors, such as age, renal function, liver function, and the presence of other medications, can influence the pharmacokinetics of IFNα.

3. Clinical uses

- Interferon-alpha (IFNα) has a wide range of clinical uses, mainly due to its immunomodulatory and antiviral properties. here are some of its primary clinical uses:
- Viral Infections: IFNα is used to treat chronic hepatitis B and hepatitis C infections, where it helps suppress viral replication and reduce liver inflammation. It is also used in some cases of chronic hepatitis D infection.
- Cancers: IFNα is used in the treatment of certain types of cancers, including hairy cell leukemia, chronic myeloid leukemia, and melanoma. It exerts its antitumor effects by inhibiting cancer cell growth and enhancing the body's immune response against cancer cells.
- Autoimmune Disorders: IFNα is used in certain autoimmune disorders, such as multiple sclerosis and systemic lupus erythematosus, to help regulate the immune response and reduce disease activity.
- Viral Warts: IFNα is used topically to treat certain types of viral warts, such as condyloma acuminatum, by stimulating the immune system to attack the wart-infected cells.
- Ocular Disorders: IFNα is used in the treatment of certain ocular disorders, such as cytomegalovirus retinitis in immunocompromised individuals.
- Hemangiomas: IFNα may be used in the treatment of certain vascular tumors, such as infantile hemangiomas, by inducing regression of the abnormal blood vessels.
- Kaposi's Sarcoma: IFNα may be used to treat Kaposi's sarcoma, a cancer often associated with immunosuppression, in some cases.

4. Toxicity

➤ Toxic effects of IFNα include GI irritation, a flulike syndrome, neutropenia, profound fatigue and myalgia, alopecia, reversible hearing loss, thyroid elimination of IFNα is mainly via proteolytic hydrolysis in the kidney. Conventional forms of IFNα are usually administered daily or 3 times a week. Pegylated forms of IFNα conjugated to polyethylene glycol can be administered once a week.

3. Clinical uses

➤ Interferonα is used in chronic HBV as an individual agent or in combination with other drugs. When used in combination with ribavirin, the progression of acute HCV infection to chronic HCV is reduced. Pegylated IFNα together with ribavirin is superior to standard forms of IFNα in chronic HCV. Other uses of IFNα include treatment of Kaposi's sarcoma, papillomatosis, and topically for genital warts.

4. Toxicity

➤ Toxic effects of IFNα include GI irritation, a flulike syndrome, neutropenia, profound fatigue and myalgia, alopecia, reversible hearing loss, thyroid dysfunction, mental confusion, and severe depression. Contraindications include pregnancy.

B. Adefovir Dipivoxil

Adefovir dipivoxil is an antiviral medication used in the treatment of chronic hepatitis B virus (HBV) infection. It is an oral prodrug of adefovir, which is a nucleotide analog. Adefovir dipivoxil is converted into its active form, adefovir, after oral administration.

Mechanism of Action:

Adefovir is a nucleotide analog that inhibits the viral DNA polymerase enzyme of hepatitis B virus. By incorporating itself into the growing viral DNA chain, it disrupts viral DNA replication and inhibits the synthesis of new viral DNA. This action helps reduce the viral load in the body, leading to a decrease in liver inflammation and improved liver function.

Clinical Uses:

Adefovir dipivoxil is primarily indicated for the treatment of chronic hepatitis B in patients with evidence of viral replication and liver inflammation. It can be used in both treatment-naive patients and those with resistance to other antiviral drugs.

It's important to note that while adefovir dipivoxil is effective in suppressing viral replication, it may not lead to complete viral eradication (a functional cure) in most patients. Therefore, long-term therapy or combination therapy with other antiviral agents may be necessary to achieve optimal treatment outcomes and prevent the development of drug resistance.

C. Entecavir

Entecavir is an antiviral medication used for the treatment of chronic hepatitis B virus (HBV) infection. It is a nucleoside analog, and its active form is incorporated into the growing viral DNA chain, disrupting viral DNA replication and inhibiting the synthesis of new viral DNA.

Mechanism of Action:

Entecavir works by selectively inhibiting the viral DNA polymerase enzyme of hepatitis B virus. By acting as a nucleoside analog, it competes with the natural building blocks (nucleotides) required for viral DNA synthesis. This results in the termination of viral DNA replication and reduces the viral load in the body.

Clinical Uses:

Entecavir is primarily indicated for the treatment of chronic hepatitis B in both treatment-naive patients and those with evidence of viral replication and liver inflammation. It is effective in suppressing viral replication and improving liver function.

Entecavir is known for its potent antiviral activity and a high barrier to resistance, meaning that it has a lower likelihood of developing drug resistance compared to some other antiviral drugs used in the treatment of HBV.

Dosage and Administration:

Entecavir is available as an oral tablet and is usually taken once daily. The dosage may vary depending on the patient's kidney function and whether they have experienced previous treatment with other antiviral agents.

Safety Considerations:

As with any medication, entecavir can have side effects, and its use should be monitored by a healthcare professional. Common side effects may include headache, fatigue, and dizziness. Patients with pre-existing kidney impairment may need dosage adjustments or closer monitoring while taking entecavir.

D. Lamivudine

Lamivudine is an antiviral medication used in the treatment of various viral infections, most notably chronic hepatitis B virus (HBV) infection and human immunodeficiency virus (HIV) infection. It is a nucleoside analog, and its active form is incorporated into the growing viral DNA or RNA chain, disrupting viral replication and inhibiting the synthesis of new viral genetic material.

Mechanism of Action:

In the context of chronic hepatitis B, lamivudine inhibits the viral reverse transcriptase enzyme of HBV. It competes with the natural building blocks (nucleotides) required for viral DNA synthesis, leading to the termination of viral DNA replication and reduction in viral load.

In the context of HIV infection, lamivudine acts as a nucleoside reverse transcriptase inhibitor (NRTI), blocking the action of HIV's reverse transcriptase enzyme. By interfering with the transcription of viral RNA into DNA, it helps inhibit viral replication and the spread of HIV in the body.

Clinical Uses:

Lamivudine is primarily indicated for the treatment of chronic hepatitis B in both treatment-naive patients and those with evidence of viral replication and liver inflammation. It is also used in the treatment of HIV infection as part of combination antiretroviral therapy to control HIV replication and delay disease progression.

Lamivudine is known for its efficacy in reducing viral replication and improving liver function in chronic hepatitis B. However, long-term monotherapy with lamivudine in chronic hepatitis B may be associated with the development of drug-resistant HBV strains over time. Therefore, it is often used in combination with other antiviral agents to achieve optimal treatment outcomes and prevent the emergence of drug resistance.

Dosage and Administration:

Lamivudine is available as an oral tablet or solution and is usually taken once daily. The dosage may vary depending on the patient's age, weight, and kidney function.

Safety Considerations:

As with any medication, lamivudine can have side effects, and its use should be monitored by a healthcare professional. Common side effects may include headache, nausea, and fatigue. Patients with pre-existing kidney impairment may need dosage adjustments or closer monitoring while taking lamivudine.

E. Ribavirin

Ribavirin is an antiviral medication used in the treatment of several viral infections, including chronic hepatitis C virus (HCV) infection and certain respiratory viral infections, such as respiratory syncytial virus (RSV) infection. It is a synthetic nucleoside analog with broad antiviral activity.

Mechanism of Action:

The exact mechanism of ribavirin's antiviral activity is not fully understood, but it is believed to have multiple effects on viral replication. Ribavirin can interfere with viral RNA synthesis, inhibit viral protein synthesis, and affect viral genome mutagenesis. These actions collectively help to reduce viral replication and inhibit the spread of the virus.

Clinical Uses:

Chronic Hepatitis C: Ribavirin is used in combination with other direct-acting antiviral agents (DAAs) for the treatment of chronic hepatitis C infection. The combination therapy with DAAs improves treatment efficacy and leads to higher cure rates (sustained virological response) compared to ribavirin monotherapy.

Respiratory Syncytial Virus (RSV) Infection: Ribavirin is used as an aerosolized formulation for the treatment of severe RSV infection in immunocompromised patients or those with severe lower respiratory tract infections.

Ribavirin is not typically used as a standalone treatment for viral infections, except in certain cases where it may be used in combination with other antiviral agents.

Dosage and Administration:

The dosage of ribavirin can vary depending on the viral infection being treated and the patient's characteristics, such as weight and kidney function. It can be administered orally or as an aerosol for inhalation.

Safety Considerations:

Ribavirin can have significant side effects, and its use should be closely monitored by a healthcare professional. Common side effects may include anemia, fatigue, headache, and rash. Ribavirin can cause hemolytic anemia (destruction of red blood cells), particularly in patients with certain conditions such as thalassemia or hemoglobinopathies. Close monitoring of hemoglobin levels is necessary during treatment.

F. Newer Drugs for HBV

Monotherapy with ribavirin alone is not effective. Early intravenous administration of ribavirin decreases mortality in viral hemorrhagic fevers. Despite its alleged activity against RSV, ribavirin has been shown to have no benefit in treatment of RSV infections, although it is still recommended by some authorities in immunocompromised children.

3. Toxicity

Systemic use results in dosedependent hemolytic anemia. Aerosol ribavirin may cause conjunctival and bronchial irritation. Ribavirin is a known human teratogen and is absolutely contraindicated in pregnancy.

F. Newer Drugs for HBV

Telbivudine, a nucleoside analog, is phosphorylated by cellular kinases to the triphosphate form, which inhibits HBV DNA polymerase. The drug is atleast as effective as lamivudine in chronic HBV infections and is similar in terms of its safety profile. Tenofovir, an antiretroviral drug, is also approved for chronic HBV infection and is active against lamivudineand entecavirresistant strains. Sofosbuvir inhibits RNA polymerase in HCV, alone or in combination with interferon or ribavirin and achieves very high cure rates (90–95%). Boceprevir is a protease inhibitor in HCV and is used in combination with ribavirin.

G. Treatment of Hepatitis C Infection

Antiviral drugs used for the treatment of Hepatitis C infection. These drugs are known as direct-acting antivirals (DAAs) and have revolutionized the management of Hepatitis C, leading to significantly improved cure rates. The four classes of DAAs are as follows:

NS3/4A Protease Inhibitors:

- Examples: Glecaprevir, Grazoprevir, Paritaprevir, Simeprevir, Voxilaprevir
- Mode of Action: NS3/4A protease inhibitors block an essential viral enzyme (NS3/4A protease), which is responsible for cleaving viral polyprotein into individual functional proteins. Inhibition of this enzyme prevents viral replication and assembly.

NS5A Inhibitors:

- Examples: Daclatasvir, Elbasvir, Ledipasvir, Ombitasvir, Pibrentasvir, Velpatasvir
- Mode of Action: NS5A inhibitors target the NS5A protein, which plays a crucial role in viral replication and assembly. By inhibiting NS5A, these drugs disrupt the viral life cycle and prevent the production of new virus particles.

NS5B Polymerase Inhibitors:

- Examples: Sofosbuvir, Dasabuvir
- Mode of Action: NS5B polymerase inhibitors interfere with the viral RNA-dependent RNA polymerase, which is essential for replicating the viral genome. By inhibiting this enzyme, the drugs block viral replication and propagation.

NS5A/NS5B Inhibitors (Combination Drugs):

➢ Examples: Epclusa (Sofosbuvir/Velpatasvir), Mavyret (Glecaprevir/Pibrentasvir)

➢ Mode of Action: Combination drugs containing both NS5A and NS5B inhibitors offer a broader antiviral activity, targeting multiple steps in the Hepatitis C virus life cycle. They improve treatment efficacy and are effective against various Hepatitis C virus genotypes.

Treatment Regimens:

Treatment regimens for Hepatitis C infection typically involve a combination of DAAs tailored to the patient's specific viral genotype, previous treatment history, and overall health status. These regimens are typically administered for 8 to 12 weeks, but the duration may vary based on individual factors. It's important to note that treatment for Hepatitis C should always be prescribed and managed by a healthcare professional with expertise in the management of viral hepatitis. Successful treatment with DAAs can result in sustained virological response (SVR), which indicates that the virus has been eradicated from the body, leading to improved liver health and a reduced risk of complications associated with chronic Hepatitis C infection.

Here is a list of common antiviral drugs used in the treatment of viral hepatitis, specifically hepatitis B and C, in a table 12t:

Hepatitis B Virus (HBV) Medications:

Drug Name	Brand Names	Type of Hepatitis B	Mechanism of Action
Entecavir	Baraclude	Hepatitis B	Nucleoside/nucleotide analog
Tenofovir disoproxil fumarate	Viread, others	Hepatitis B	Nucleoside/nucleotide analog
Tenofovir alafenamide	Vemlidy	Hepatitis B	Nucleoside/nucleotide analog
Lamivudine	Epivir-HBV	Hepatitis B	Nucleoside/nucleotide analog

| Adefovir dipivoxil | Hepsera | Hepatitis B | Nucleoside/nucleotide analog |
| Interferon alfa-2b | Intron A, others | Hepatitis B | Immunomodulatory |

Hepatitis C Virus (HCV) Medications: table 12.1

Drug Name	Brand Names	Type of Hepatitis C	Mechanism of Action
Sofosbuvir	Sovaldi	Hepatitis C (all genotypes)	Direct-acting antiviral (DAA)
Ledipasvir/sofosbuvir	Harvoni	Hepatitis C (genotype 1)	DAA combination
Daclatasvir	Daklinza	Hepatitis C (genotype 3)	DAA
Ombitasvir/paritaprevir/ritonavir	Technivie	Hepatitis C (genotype 4)	DAA combination
Elbasvir/grazoprevir	Zepatier	Hepatitis C (genotype 1, 4)	DAA combination
Velpatasvir/sofosbuvir	Epclusa	Hepatitis C (all genotypes)	DAA combination
Glecaprevir/pibrentasvir	Mavyret	Hepatitis C (all genotypes)	DAA combination
Ribavirin	Copegus, others	Hepatitis C (used in combination)	Nucleoside analog
Peginterferon alfa-2a	Pegasys	Hepatitis C (used in combination)	Immunomodulatory

Please note that treatment for viral hepatitis can be complex and typically involves a combination of antiviral medications, often tailored to the specific genotype of the virus, the patient's medical history, and other factors. The introduction of direct-acting antivirals (DAAs) has revolutionized the treatment of hepatitis C, leading to higher cure rates and shorter treatment durations.

CHECKLIST

When you complete this chapter, you should be able to:

- Identify the main targets for antiviral action in viral replication.
- Describe the mechanisms of action of antiherpes drugs and the mechanisms of HSV and CMV resistance.
- List the main pharmacokinetic properties and toxic effects of acyclovir, ganciclovir, cidofovir, and foscarnet.
- Describe the mechanisms of antiHIV
- action of zidovudine, indinavir, and enfuvirtide.
- Match a specific antiretroviral drug with each of the following: to be avoided in pregnancy; hyperpigmentation; neutropenia; pancreatitis;
- peripheral neuropathy; inhibition of P450; severe hypersensitivity reaction; injection site reactions.
- Identify the significant properties of 4 drugs active against HBV and HCV.
- Identify the significant properties of an antiinfluenza
- drug acting at the stage of viral uncoating and another acting at the stage of viral release

(Anderson et al., 2009)

Targets / Strategies	Enzymes / Mechanisms	Antiviral Drugs	Viruses
Viral enzymes	Polymerase	Acyclovir, Ganciclovir, Penciclovir,	Herpes viruses
		Lamivudine, Adefovir, Entecavir,	HBV
		Valopicitabine	HCV
	Protease	Amprenavir, Atazanavir, Ritonavir, Tipranavir	HIV
		VX-950	HCV
	Neuraminidase	Oseltamivir, Zanamivir	Influenza virus
Cellular targets	Receptors or co-receptors	Maraviroc, *Vicriviroc, TNX-355, Pro-140*	HIV
	Capping enzyme	Ribavirin	HCV
	Immune response	Interferons	HBV, HCV
		Actilon	HCV
Other viral targets	*Attachment proteins*	BMS-488043	*HIV*
	Fusion proteins	Enfuvirtide	HIV
	Disassembly/Uncoating	Amantadine, Rimantadine *Pleconaril*	Influenza virus, *Picornaviruses*
	Virion maturation	Bevirimat UK-201844	HIV
Novel strategies	Antisense RNA *Ribozymes*	Fomivirsen	CMV retinitis

DRUGS ACTING ON CLOTTING DISORDERS

Anticoagulants drugs.

Anticoagulant drugs can be classified into different categories based on their mechanisms of action and clinical uses. Here are some common classifications of anticoagulant drugs:

Vitamin K Antagonists:

These drugs interfere with the body's use of vitamin K, which is necessary for the production of clotting factors.

Example: Warfarin (Coumadin)

Heparins:

Heparins are natural anticoagulants that work by enhancing the activity of antithrombin III, a protein that inhibits clot formation.

Examples: Unfractionated heparin (UFH), Low Molecular Weight Heparins (LMWHs) such as enoxaparin (Lovenox) and dalteparin (Fragmin).

Direct Oral Anticoagulants (DOACs) / Novel Oral Anticoagulants (NOACs):

DOACs act directly on specific clotting factors and do not require frequent monitoring.

Subcategories include:

Direct Thrombin Inhibitors: Example - Dabigatran (Pradaxa).

Factor Xa Inhibitors: Examples - Rivaroxaban (Xarelto), Apixaban (Eliquis), Edoxaban (Savaysa).

Antiplatelet Agents:

These drugs prevent platelets from sticking together and forming clots.

Examples: Aspirin, Clopidogrel (Plavix), Prasugrel (Effient), Ticagrelor (Brilinta).

Thrombolytics (Fibrinolytics):

Thrombolytics are used to dissolve existing blood clots.

Example: Alteplase (tPA), Streptokinase.

Other Anticoagulants:

This category includes anticoagulants that don't fit into the above classifications.

Examples: Fondaparinux (Arixtra), Bivalirudin (Angiomax), Argatroban.

Oral Anticoagulants (Coumarins):

These are a subset of vitamin K antagonists.

Example: Acenocoumarol.

Anti-Xa Inhibitors:

These drugs specifically inhibit factor Xa, a key enzyme in the blood clotting cascade.

Examples: Rivaroxaban, Apixaban.

Anti-IIa Inhibitors:

These drugs inhibit thrombin, another key enzyme in the clotting cascade.

Example: Dabigatran.

Vitamin K Antagonists:

Mechanism of Action:

Vitamin K antagonists, such as warfarin, act by interfering with the body's use of vitamin K, which is essential for the production of clotting factors. They inhibit the enzymes responsible for activating clotting factors II (prothrombin), VII, IX, and X, as well as proteins C and S. By inhibiting these clotting factors, vitamin K antagonists slow down the blood clotting process, making it harder for clots to form.

Pharmacokinetics:

- Absorption: Warfarin is administered orally and is well-absorbed from the gastrointestinal tract.
- Distribution: It is highly protein-bound to albumin in the plasma, and this binding can be affected by other drugs.
- Metabolism: Warfarin undergoes extensive metabolism in the liver through the cytochrome P450 system.
- Excretion: Metabolites are excreted primarily in the urine and, to a lesser extent, in the feces.

Therapeutic Uses:

- Vitamin K antagonists are primarily used for their anticoagulant properties to prevent and treat conditions associated with blood clot formation, such as:
- Venous Thromboembolism (VTE): Including deep vein thrombosis (DVT) and pulmonary embolism (PE).
- Atrial Fibrillation: To reduce the risk of stroke by preventing the formation of atrial blood clots.
- Prosthetic Heart Valves: Preventing clot formation on mechanical heart valves.
- Myocardial Infarction (MI): As part of long-term therapy to reduce the risk of recurrent events.

Adverse Effects:

- Bleeding: The primary concern with vitamin K antagonists is the risk of bleeding, which can range from minor nosebleeds to life-threatening bleeding events.
- Hemorrhagic Stroke: Excessive anticoagulation can lead to bleeding within the brain, resulting in a hemorrhagic stroke.

- Skin Necrosis: A rare complication that may occur when therapy is initiated, especially in protein C-deficient patients
- Drug Interactions: Vitamin K antagonists interact with many drugs and dietary factors that can affect their anticoagulant effect. Regular monitoring is required to maintain the desired level of anticoagulation.

Heparins:

Mechanism of Action:

Heparins are a class of anticoagulant drugs that primarily work by enhancing the activity of antithrombin III, a natural anticoagulant in the body. Antithrombin III inhibits several clotting factors, including thrombin (factor IIa) and factor Xa. Heparins bind to antithrombin III and enhance its inhibitory effect on these clotting factors, preventing the formation of blood clots.

Pharmacokinetics:

- The pharmacokinetics of heparins can vary depending on whether they are administered subcutaneously or intravenously:
- Subcutaneous Heparins: These are generally well-absorbed after subcutaneous injection.
- Intravenous Heparins: When administered intravenously, heparins have an immediate onset of action, as they directly affect circulating blood.
- Heparins have a relatively short half-life, which allows for quick reversibility if necessary.

Therapeutic Uses:

- Heparins are used for various therapeutic purposes related to their anticoagulant properties, such as:
- Deep Vein Thrombosis (DVT) and Pulmonary Embolism (PE): Heparins are used for the initial treatment of DVT and PE to prevent further clot formation.
- Prophylaxis: They are used to prevent the formation of clots in patients at risk of DVT, such as those undergoing surgery or bedridden individuals.

- Acute Coronary Syndromes: Heparins are used in combination with antiplatelet agents in the management of conditions like unstable angina and non-ST-segment elevation myocardial infarction.
- Cardiopulmonary Bypass: Heparins are used during open-heart surgery to prevent clot formation within the heart-lung machine.

Adverse Effects:

- Bleeding: Like other anticoagulants, heparins can lead to bleeding, which can range from mild to severe.
- Heparin-Induced Thrombocytopenia (HIT): A rare but serious side effect characterized by a drop in platelet count and an increased risk of clot formation.
- Osteoporosis: Long-term use of heparins can lead to decreased bone density, increasing the risk of fractures.
- Hypersensitivity Reactions: Allergic reactions to heparins are rare but can occur.
- Alopecia (Hair Loss): Occasional reports of hair loss have been associated with the use of heparins.

Direct Oral Anticoagulants (DOACs) / Novel Oral Anticoagulants (NOACs):

Mechanism of Action:

- Direct Oral Anticoagulants (DOACs), also known as Novel Oral Anticoagulants (NOACs), work by targeting specific clotting factors in the blood. There are different types of DOACs, each with a unique mechanism of action:
- Direct Thrombin Inhibitors: Examples include dabigatran. They directly inhibit thrombin (factor IIa), a key enzyme in the coagulation cascade.
- Factor Xa Inhibitors: Examples include apixaban, rivaroxaban, edoxaban, and betrixaban. These drugs specifically target factor Xa, which plays a crucial role in blood clot formation.
- DOACs interfere with these specific clotting factors to prevent the formation of blood clots. Unlike traditional anticoagulants like heparins and vitamin K

antagonists, DOACs work more selectively, which can simplify dosing and monitoring.

Pharmacokinetics:

The pharmacokinetics of DOACs can vary by the specific drug, but they generally exhibit the following characteristics: Rapid onset of action, Predictable pharmacokinetics, reducing the need for frequent monitoring. Many DOACs have relatively short half-lives.

Therapeutic Uses:

DOACs are used for various therapeutic purposes related to their anticoagulant properties:

1. Prevention and Treatment of Deep Vein Thrombosis (DVT) and Pulmonary Embolism (PE): DOACs are used for the prevention and treatment of DVT and PE.
2. Stroke Prevention in Atrial Fibrillation: They are commonly used to reduce the risk of stroke and systemic embolism in patients with atrial fibrillation.
3. Venous Thromboembolism (VTE) Prophylaxis: DOACs may be prescribed to prevent VTE after major orthopedic surgeries.
4. Treatment of VTE: They are also used for the treatment of acute VTE, including DVT and PE.

Adverse Effects:
- While DOACs have several advantages over traditional anticoagulants, they are not without side effects or potential adverse events:
- *Bleeding*: The most common adverse effect is bleeding. Although DOACs have a lower risk of intracranial bleeding compared to warfarin, they can still lead to significant bleeding events.
- *Gastrointestinal Disturbances*: Some patients may experience gastrointestinal symptoms like upset stomach or diarrhea.
- *Renal Impairment*: Dosing adjustments are often required for individuals with impaired kidney function.
- *Liver Enzyme Elevations*: Elevated liver enzymes can occur in some cases.
- *Allergic Reactions*: Allergic reactions to DOACs are rare but possible.

ANTIBIOTICS

Antibiotics are chemotherapeutic drugs of biological nature inhibiting microorganism selectively.

Antibiotics are divided according chemical structure:

1. Beta-lactam antibiotics (penicillins, cefalosporins, monobactams, carbopenems);

2. Macrolides and azalidesl

3. Aminoglycosides;

4. Tetracyclines;

5. Laevomycetines;

6. Polyenes;

7. Glycopeptide antibiotics;

8. Lincosamides;

9. Polymyxines;

10. Steroid structure antibiotics;

11. Antibiotics of different chemical groups.

Classification according to mechanism of action:

Antibiotics can be classified based on their mechanism of action. Here are some common classes of antibiotics and their mechanisms:

Cell Wall Synthesis Inhibitors:

- Beta-Lactam Antibiotics: These include penicillins, cephalosporins, carbapenems, and monobactams. They inhibit the synthesis of bacterial cell walls by targeting enzymes involved in peptidoglycan formation.
- Glycopeptides: An example is vancomycin, which disrupts cell wall synthesis in Gram-positive bacteria.

Protein Synthesis Inhibitors:

- Aminoglycosides: Such as gentamicin and streptomycin. They interfere with protein synthesis by binding to the bacterial ribosome.
- Tetracyclines: Like doxycycline, they block protein synthesis by preventing tRNA from binding to the ribosome.
- Macrolides: Erythromycin and azithromycin inhibit protein synthesis by blocking the bacterial ribosome.
- Chloramphenicol: It inhibits protein synthesis by interfering with the ribosome.
- Oxazolidinones: Linezolid is an example that inhibits protein synthesis.

Nucleic Acid Synthesis Inhibitors:

- Quinolones: Ciprofloxacin and levofloxacin interfere with DNA synthesis by targeting DNA gyrase and topoisomerase IV.
- Rifamycins: Rifampin inhibits RNA synthesis in bacteria.
- Metabolic Pathway Inhibitors:
- Sulfonamides: Like sulfamethoxazole, they block the synthesis of folic acid, an essential cofactor for nucleic acid and amino acid synthesis.
- Trimethoprim: It inhibits the same folic acid pathway.

Cell Membrane Disruptors:

- Polymyxins: Polymyxin B and colistin disrupt the cell membrane of Gram-negative bacteria.
- Antibiotics with Unique Mechanisms:
- Daptomycin: It disrupts bacterial cell membrane function by forming pores.
- Fosfomycin: It inhibits bacterial cell wall synthesis.

Anti-Tuberculosis Agents:
- Isoniazid: Targets mycobacterial cell wall synthesis.
- Ethambutol: Inhibits mycobacterial cell wall synthesis.
- Antifungals:
- Azoles: Fluconazole and voriconazole inhibit fungal ergosterol synthesis.
- Polyenes: Amphotericin B disrupts fungal cell membranes.
- Echinocandins: Caspofungin inhibits fungal cell wall synthesis.

Antiviral Agents:
- Nucleoside/Nucleotide Analogs: Antivirals like acyclovir, tenofovir, and zidovudine interfere with viral replication by targeting nucleic acid synthesis.
- Protease Inhibitors: Examples include ritonavir and lopinavir. They block viral proteases involved in viral replication.
- Neuraminidase Inhibitors: Oseltamivir and zanamivir inhibit neuraminidase in influenza viruses.

Classification according to the spectrum of action:

Antibiotics can also be classified based on their spectrum of action, which refers to the range of bacteria against which they are effective. There are two primary categories:

Broad-Spectrum Antibiotics:
- These antibiotics are effective against a wide range of bacteria, both Gram-positive and Gram-negative.
- They are often used when the infecting organism is not known or when the infection involves multiple types of bacteria.
- Examples include:
- Ampicillin and Amoxicillin: Effective against many Gram-positive and Gram-negative bacteria.
- Ciprofloxacin: Effective against a broad range of bacteria, including those causing urinary tract infections.

- Tetracyclines: Active against various bacteria, both Gram-positive and Gram-negative.

Narrow-Spectrum Antibiotics:

- These antibiotics target a specific group of bacteria, typically either Gram-positive or Gram-negative bacteria.
- They are often chosen when the infecting organism is known, and a more targeted approach is desired to reduce the risk of antibiotic resistance.

Examples include:

- Penicillin G: Effective primarily against Gram-positive bacteria, such as Streptococcus and Staphylococcus.
- Cefazolin: Used for surgical prophylaxis against Gram-positive bacteria.
- Vancomycin: Active against Gram-positive bacteria and often used for severe infections like MRSA.
- Polymyxin B: Effective against Gram-negative bacteria, especially Pseudomonas.

Extended-Spectrum Antibiotics:

- These antibiotics have an intermediate spectrum of action, covering a broader range than narrow-spectrum antibiotics but not as wide as broad-spectrum antibiotics.
- They may be used when a specific range of bacteria is suspected but not confirmed.

Examples include:

- Piperacillin/Tazobactam: Effective against Gram-negative and some Gram-positive bacteria.
- Amoxicillin/Clavulanic Acid (Augmentin): Effective against both Gram-positive and Gram-negative bacteria.

List of Antibiotic Class, examples of antibiotic drugs and their mode of action in Table 13

Antibiotic Class	Examples of Antibiotics	Mode of Action
Penicillins	Amoxicillin, Ampicillin, Penicillin G	Inhibit bacterial cell wall synthesis
Cephalosporins	Cephalexin, Ceftriaxone, Cefuroxime	Inhibit bacterial cell wall synthesis
Carbapenems	Imipenem, Meropenem, Doripenem	Inhibit bacterial cell wall synthesis
Monobactams	Aztreonam	Inhibit bacterial cell wall synthesis
Aminoglycosides	Gentamicin, Tobramycin, Amikacin	Inhibit bacterial protein synthesis
Tetracyclines	Doxycycline, Tetracycline, Minocycline	Inhibit bacterial protein synthesis
Macrolides	Azithromycin, Clarithromycin, Erythromycin	Inhibit bacterial protein synthesis
Lincosamides	Clindamycin	Inhibit bacterial protein synthesis
Sulfonamides	Sulfamethoxazole, Trimethoprim-Sulfamethoxazole (Co-trimoxazole)	Inhibit bacterial folic acid synthesis
Quinolones (Fluoroquinolones)	Ciprofloxacin, Levofloxacin, Moxifloxacin	Inhibit bacterial DNA synthesis and replication
Nitrofurans	Nitrofurantoin	Damage bacterial DNA and inhibit RNA synthesis
Metronidazoles	Metronidazole	Disrupt bacterial DNA and inhibit nucleic acid synthesis
Glycopeptides	Vancomycin, Teicoplanin	Inhibit bacterial cell wall synthesis

Oxazolidinones	Linezolid	Inhibit bacterial protein synthesis
Lipopeptides	Daptomycin	Disrupt bacterial cell membrane

Penicillins

Classification of Penicillins Table 14

Classification of Penicillins	Examples	Characteristics
Natural Penicillins	Penicillin G (Benzylpenicillin)	Effective against Gram-positive bacteria.
	Penicillin V	Often administered orally.
Aminopenicillins	Amoxicillin	Broader spectrum against Gram-negative bacteria, including some Enterobacteriaceae.
	Ampicillin	Similar spectrum to amoxicillin.
Antistaphylococcal Penicillins	Methicillin	Effective against Staphylococcus aureus, including some resistant strains.
	Oxacillin	Also used against Staphylococcus aureus, including methicillin-resistant strains.
Extended-Spectrum Penicillins	Piperacillin	Effective against a wider range of Gram-negative bacteria, including Pseudomonas.
	Ticarcillin	Similar to piperacillin, used in combination with beta-lactamase inhibitors.

Natural Penicillins:

Mechanism of Action:

Natural penicillins, such as penicillin G and penicillin V, work by inhibiting the synthesis of the bacterial cell wall. They do this by binding to and inhibiting an enzyme called transpeptidase (penicillin-binding protein), which is involved in cross-linking the peptidoglycan chains in the cell wall. This action weakens the bacterial cell wall, making it susceptible to osmotic lysis, ultimately leading to bacterial cell death.

Pharmacokinetics:

- Natural penicillins are typically administered via intravenous (IV) or intramuscular (IM) injection as penicillin G or orally as penicillin V.
- They are absorbed from the gastrointestinal tract after oral administration.
- These drugs have a short half-life and are eliminated primarily through renal excretion.

Therapeutic Uses:

- Natural penicillins are effective against a wide range of Gram-positive bacteria, including Streptococcus, Staphylococcus, and Enterococcus species.
- They are commonly used to treat various infections, such as streptococcal infections (e.g., strep throat), skin and soft tissue infections, syphilis, and endocarditis.

Adverse Effects:

- Common side effects may include allergic reactions, including skin rashes and hives.
- Anaphylaxis, a severe allergic reaction, can occur rarely and is a medical emergency.
- Gastrointestinal disturbances like nausea, vomiting, and diarrhea can occur.
- Neurological side effects are possible, including seizures (more common with high doses).
- Hypokalemia (low blood potassium levels) may occur.

Cephalosporins

Cephalosporins are a class of antibiotics that are structurally related to penicillins. They are categorized into generations based on their spectrum of activity and mechanisms of action. Here's a classification of cephalosporins with their respective mechanisms of action: Table 14

Generation	Examples	Mechanism of Action
First Generation	Cefazolin, Cephalexin	Mechanism of Action: - Inhibit cell wall synthesis by binding to penicillin-binding proteins (PBPs) in bacterial cell walls. - Disrupt peptidoglycan cross-linking, leading to cell wall weakening and bacterial cell lysis.
Second Generation	Cefuroxime, Cefoxitin	Mechanism of Action: - Similar to first-generation cephalosporins, they inhibit cell wall synthesis by binding to PBPs. - Extended spectrum of activity against Gram-negative bacteria compared to first-generation drugs.
Third Generation	Ceftriaxone, Cefotaxime	Mechanism of Action: - Extended activity against Gram-negative bacteria, especially Enterobacteriaceae. - High affinity for PBPs, leading to inhibition of cell wall synthesis.
Fourth Generation	Cefepime	Mechanism of Action: - Broader spectrum, including both Gram-positive and Gram-negative bacteria. - Inhibition of cell wall synthesis by binding to PBPs.
Fifth Generation	Ceftaroline	Mechanism of Action: - Enhanced activity against Gram-positive bacteria, including methicillin-resistant Staphylococcus aureus (MRSA). - Inhibition of cell wall synthesis.

Adverse effects associated with cephalosporins can vary depending on the specific drug within the cephalosporin class and an individual's response. However, there are some common adverse effects that can occur with cephalosporin antibiotics:

Gastrointestinal Effects:

- Nausea
- Vomiting
- Diarrhea
- Abdominal pain or discomfort

Hypersensitivity Reactions:

- Allergic reactions ranging from mild skin rashes to severe anaphylaxis (a life-threatening reaction)
- Cross-reactivity with penicillin allergy is possible, although it occurs less frequently than in the past.

Superinfections:

- Use of cephalosporins can lead to the overgrowth of non-susceptible microorganisms, such as Clostridium difficile, leading to antibiotic-associated colitis or diarrhea.

Renal Effects:

- Occasionally, cephalosporins can affect kidney function, leading to kidney problems.

Hematologic Effects:

- Rarely, cephalosporins can cause blood disorders, including a decrease in white blood cell count (leukopenia) and a decrease in platelets (thrombocytopenia).

Neurological Effects:

- High doses or prolonged use of cephalosporins may lead to neurological symptoms, such as seizures.

Hepatic Effects:

- Cephalosporins can sometimes cause liver function abnormalities.

Local Reactions:

- Pain, inflammation, or thrombophlebitis at the injection site for intravenous formulations.

Moxalactam

Moxalactam is a broad-spectrum antibiotic that belongs to the cephalosporin class. It was once widely used to treat various bacterial infections, but its use has become less common over the years. This antibiotic is notable for its effectiveness against a wide range of both Gram-positive and Gram-negative bacteria. Moxalactam works by interfering with the synthesis of bacterial cell walls, ultimately leading to bacterial cell death.

Moxalactam was particularly useful in treating infections that were resistant to other antibiotics. However, due to the development of newer antibiotics and the occurrence of bacterial resistance to moxalactam itself, its use has declined. Despite its reduced usage, moxalactam remains an important part of the history of antibiotic development and the fight against bacterial infections. Table 15

Classification	Moxalactam
Mechanism of Action	Moxalactam is a beta-lactam antibiotic that inhibits bacterial cell wall synthesis by binding to penicillin-binding proteins (PBPs). It disrupts peptidoglycan cross-link formation, weakening the bacterial cell wall and leading to cell lysis. It has a broad spectrum of activity, effective against various Gram-negative and some Gram-positive bacteria.
Therapeutic Uses	Moxalactam is used to treat a wide range of infections caused by susceptible bacteria, including urinary tract infections, respiratory tract infections, intra-abdominal infections, skin and soft tissue infections, and gynecological infections. It is particularly effective against beta-lactamase-producing bacteria.
Adverse Effects	Common adverse effects may include gastrointestinal symptoms (nausea, diarrhea), skin rashes, and hypersensitivity reactions. As with other antibiotics, there's a risk of developing Clostridium difficile-associated diarrhea. Moxalactam may also cause pain and inflammation at the injection site. Serious but rare adverse effects include severe allergic reactions, blood disorders, and kidney problems. It's important to report any unusual or severe side effects to a healthcare provider.

Monobactams

Table 16 Classification of monobactum their therapeutic use and Adverse effects

Classification	Mechanism of Action	Therapeutic Uses	Adverse Effects
Second-generation cephalosporin	Inhibits bacterial cell wall synthesis by binding to penicillin-binding proteins (PBPs).	Used to treat a wide range of bacterial infections, including respiratory, urinary tract, skin, and soft tissue infections.	Common side effects: gastrointestinal issues (nausea, vomiting, diarrhea), skin rashes, allergic reactions. May lead to superinfections.

Aminoglycosides

The aminoglycosides are compounds containing characteristics amino sugars joined to a hexose nucleus in glycosidic linkage. They are polycations and their polarity accounts for their pharmacokinetic properties. Aminoglycosides are a class of antibiotics that are primarily effective against various Gram-negative bacteria. They inhibit bacterial protein synthesis by binding to the ribosomal subunit, which leads to the production of nonfunctional or toxic peptides, ultimately killing the bacteria.

Here is a table 17 with a list of aminoglycosides, their classification, and mechanism of action:

Aminoglycoside	Classification	Mechanism of Action
Gentamicin	Aminoglycoside	Inhibits bacterial protein synthesis by binding to 30S subunit of ribosome, leading to misreading of mRNA.
Tobramycin	Aminoglycoside	Similar to gentamicin, it disrupts bacterial protein synthesis by binding to the 30S ribosomal subunit.

Amikacin	Aminoglycoside	Exerts bactericidal effects by interfering with bacterial protein synthesis, particularly against Gram-negative bacteria.

Gentamicin:

Therapeutic Uses:

- Used for severe Gram-negative bacterial infections such as Pseudomonas aeruginosa, Escherichia coli, and Klebsiella species.
- Often used in combination with other antibiotics to treat complicated infections.
- May be used to treat certain mycobacterial infections like Mycobacterium avium complex.

Adverse Effects:

- Nephrotoxicity (kidney damage)
- Ototoxicity (damage to the inner ear, affecting hearing and balance)
- Neuromuscular blockade in high doses.

Tobramycin:

Therapeutic Uses:

- Commonly used to treat respiratory infections in patients with cystic fibrosis.
- Effective against various Gram-negative bacteria, including Pseudomonas aeruginosa.

Adverse Effects:

- Nephrotoxicity
- Ototoxicity
- Neuromuscular blockade in high doses.

Amikacin:

Therapeutic Uses:
- Reserved for severe infections when other antibiotics have failed or when the infection is caused by multidrug-resistant bacteria.
- Effective against various Gram-negative bacteria.

Adverse Effects:
- Nephrotoxicity
- Ototoxicity
- Neuromuscular blockade in high doses.

Tetracyclines

Tetracyclines are broad-spectrum antibiotics that inhibit protein synthesis in bacteria by interfering with the ribosomal machinery, specifically the 30S ribosomal subunit. This action prevents the addition of amino acids to the growing peptide chain, ultimately inhibiting bacterial growth. Table 18

Tetracycline Antibiotic	Classification	Mechanism of Action
Doxycycline	Tetracycline	Inhibits bacterial protein synthesis by binding to the 30S ribosomal subunit, preventing the addition of amino acids to the growing peptide chain.
Minocycline	Tetracycline	Similar to doxycycline, it inhibits protein synthesis by binding to the 30S ribosomal subunit.
Tetracycline	Tetracycline	Acts by binding to the bacterial ribosome and interfering with protein synthesis.

Therapeutic Uses of Tetracyclines:

Infections:

1. Tetracyclines are effective against a wide range of bacterial infections, including:
   - Respiratory tract infections such as pneumonia and bronchitis.
   - Skin and soft tissue infections, like acne, cellulitis, and abscesses.
   - Sexually transmitted infections, including chlamydia, gonorrhea, and syphilis.
   - Urinary tract infections.
2. *Rickettsial Infections:* Tetracyclines are the first-line treatment for rickettsial diseases, such as Rocky Mountain spotted fever.
3. *Lyme Disease*: Doxycycline is often used to treat Lyme disease, particularly in the early stages.
4. *Malaria*: Tetracyclines, including doxycycline, are used as prophylaxis against malaria when traveling to endemic regions.
5. *Acne Vulgaris*: Tetracyclines are effective in managing moderate to severe acne, reducing inflammation and controlling the growth of acne-causing bacteria.

Adverse Effects of Tetracyclines:

1. *Gastrointestinal Distress:* Tetracyclines can cause nausea, vomiting, and diarrhea. Taking them with food or milk can help reduce stomach upset.
2. *Photosensitivity*: Tetracyclines make the skin more sensitive to sunlight, increasing the risk of sunburn. Sunscreen and protective clothing are recommended.
3. *Teeth Discoloration*: Tetracyclines can permanently discolor developing teeth in children. They should not be used in pregnant women or children under 8 years old.
4. *Hepatotoxicity:* Rare cases of liver damage have been reported, so monitoring liver function may be necessary during treatment.
5. *Renal Toxicity*: Prolonged use or high doses can affect kidney function, so adequate hydration is essential.

6. *Hypersensitivity Reactions*: Some individuals may experience allergic reactions, including skin rashes and itching.
7. *Esophageal Ulceration*: Tetracyclines can cause irritation to the esophagus, so it's essential to take them with a full glass of water and remain upright for at least 30 minutes after ingestion.
8. *Interactions:* Tetracyclines can interact with other drugs, reducing their effectiveness or causing adverse effects. It's crucial to inform your healthcare provider of all medications you are taking.

Lincosamides

Lincosamides are effective antibiotics that act by disrupting bacterial protein synthesis. They are particularly useful in treating various infections caused by anaerobic bacteria, streptococci, and some staphylococci. Table 19

Classification	Examples	Mechanism of Action
Lincosamides	Lincomycin, Clindamycin	Inhibit protein synthesis in bacteria by binding to the 50S subunit of the bacterial ribosome, which prevents the addition of new amino acids to the growing peptide chain, thereby halting protein synthesis.

Therapeutic Uses:

1. Bacterial Infections: Lincosamides are primarily used to treat various bacterial infections, including skin and soft tissue infections, bone and joint infections, and respiratory tract infections.
2. Anaerobic Infections: They are effective against anaerobic bacteria, making them suitable for treating anaerobic infections such as intra-abdominal infections and dental infections.
3. Streptococcal Infections: Lincosamides are used to manage infections caused by Streptococcal bacteria, including Streptococcus pneumoniae and Streptococcus pyogenes.
4. Pelvic Inflammatory Disease (PID): Clindamycin, a Lincosamide, is sometimes prescribed in combination with other antibiotics to treat PID.

Adverse Effects:

1. Gastrointestinal Disturbances: Common adverse effects include nausea, vomiting, diarrhea, and abdominal pain. It's advisable to take them with food to reduce stomach discomfort.
2. Clostridium difficile Infection: Lincosamides can disrupt the normal gut flora, leading to overgrowth of the bacterium Clostridium difficile, which can cause severe diarrhea and colitis.
3. Allergic Reactions: Some individuals may experience allergic reactions such as skin rashes, itching, or hives.
4. Pseudomembranous Colitis: Lincosamides, particularly Clindamycin, can increase the risk of developing pseudomembranous colitis, a severe and potentially life-threatening condition characterized by severe diarrhea and inflammation of the colon.
5. Hepatic Effects: Lincosamides may lead to abnormal liver function tests in some cases, and rarely, they can cause severe liver damage.
6. Blood Disorders: There have been reports of blood disorders like neutropenia, eosinophilia, and agranulocytosis associated with the use of Lincosamides.
7. Hypersensitivity Reactions: In rare instances, individuals may experience severe hypersensitivity reactions, including anaphylaxis, which is a medical emergency.

Sulfonamides

Sulfonamides are a class of synthetic antimicrobial drugs that work by inhibiting the bacterial enzyme dihydropteroate synthase, a key component in the synthesis of folic acid (folate). By blocking folate production, sulfonamides interfere with the ability of bacteria to synthesize DNA, RNA, and proteins. This leads to the inhibition of bacterial growth and ultimately the death of susceptible bacteria. Sulfonamides are bacteriostatic, meaning they stop the growth and reproduction of bacteria but do not necessarily kill them directly.

The effectiveness of sulfonamides can be enhanced when used in combination with other antimicrobial agents like trimethoprim (co-trimoxazole). This combination therapy is often used to treat a wide range of bacterial infections, such as urinary tract infections, respiratory tract infections, and certain types of skin infections. It is also used for the prevention and treatment of malaria caused by Plasmodium falciparum and Toxoplasma gondii. Table 20

Sulfonamide	Examples	Mechanism of Action
Short-Acting Sulfonamides	Sulfisoxazole	Inhibit bacterial dihydropteroate synthase, an enzyme involved in folate synthesis. Bacteria require folate for DNA synthesis and growth.
Intermediate-Acting Sulfonamides	Sulfamethoxazole	Similar to short-acting sulfonamides, they inhibit dihydropteroate synthase, disrupting bacterial folate synthesis. Often used in combination with trimethoprim for enhanced effect.
Long-Acting Sulfonamides	Sulfadoxine, Sulfamethoxypyridazine	Inhibit dihydropteroate synthase like other sulfonamides but have longer duration of action. Used in combination therapy for malaria.

Therapeutic Uses of Sulfonamides:

1. Bacterial Infections: Sulfonamides are effective against a wide range of bacterial infections, including urinary tract infections (UTIs), respiratory tract infections, ear infections, and eye infections.
2. Malaria: Sulfadoxine-pyrimethamine (SP) is used for both the treatment and prevention of malaria, particularly in areas with Plasmodium falciparum resistance to other antimalarial drugs.
3. Toxoplasmosis: Sulfadiazine, often in combination with pyrimethamine, is used for the treatment of toxoplasmosis, an infection caused by the parasite Toxoplasma gondii.
4. Inflammatory Bowel Disease: Sulfasalazine is used in the management of inflammatory bowel diseases, such as ulcerative colitis and Crohn's disease.
5. Burns and Wound Care: Sulfadiazine cream is applied topically to prevent or treat infections in burn wounds and other open wounds.

Adverse Effects of Sulfonamides:

1. Hypersensitivity Reactions: Sulfonamides are associated with various hypersensitivity reactions, including skin rashes, hives, and more severe reactions like Stevens-Johnson syndrome and toxic epidermal necrolysis. These reactions can be life-threatening.
2. Gastrointestinal Distress: Nausea, vomiting, diarrhea, and loss of appetite are common gastrointestinal side effects of sulfonamides.
3. Hematologic Effects: Sulfonamides can lead to blood disorders, such as hemolytic anemia, agranulocytosis (a severe reduction in white blood cells), and thrombocytopenia (reduced platelets).
4. Renal Effects: Some sulfonamides can cause crystalluria, which may lead to kidney damage or kidney stones.
5. Photosensitivity: Sulfonamides can increase sensitivity to sunlight, leading to skin reactions when exposed to UV light.
6. Liver Toxicity: Hepatotoxicity, although rare, can occur with sulfonamide use, leading to liver damage.
7. Central Nervous System Effects: Sulfonamides may cause headaches, dizziness, or altered mental status in some individuals.
8. Hypoglycemia: Sulfonamides may lead to low blood sugar levels, particularly in people with diabetes.
9. Allergic Reactions: Anaphylactic reactions, while rare, can be life-threatening and require immediate medical attention.
10. Respiratory Reactions: Sulfonamides may cause respiratory distress or bronchospasm in individuals with pre-existing respiratory conditions.

Quinolones

Quinolones work by inhibiting DNA gyrase and topoisomerase IV, which are enzymes involved in DNA replication, transcription, and repair in bacteria. This inhibition leads to the accumulation of double-stranded breaks in bacterial DNA, ultimately causing cell death. Table 21

Classification	Example Quinolones	Mechanism of Action
First Generation	Ciprofloxacin	Inhibition of DNA gyrase and topoisomerase IV, enzymes required for DNA replication and repair in bacteria.
Second Generation	Ofloxacin, Norfloxacin	Similar to first-generation quinolones, inhibiting DNA gyrase and topoisomerase IV. Second-generation drugs have an expanded spectrum of activity.
Third Generation	Levofloxacin, Sparfloxacin	Enhanced activity against both Gram-positive and Gram-negative bacteria.
Fourth Generation	Moxifloxacin, Gatifloxacin	Broader spectrum of activity, including atypical pathogens like Mycoplasma and Chlamydia, as well as enhanced activity against Gram-positive bacteria.

Therapeutic Uses:

1. Bacterial Infections: Quinolones are used to treat a wide range of bacterial infections, including urinary tract infections, respiratory tract infections, skin and soft tissue infections, and sexually transmitted infections.
2. Respiratory Infections: They are prescribed for pneumonia and bronchitis, particularly for atypical pathogens.
3. Gastrointestinal Infections: Quinolones can be effective against some gastrointestinal infections, including traveler's diarrhea.
4. Bone and Joint Infections: They may be used for chronic osteomyelitis or complicated joint infections.

5. Intra-Abdominal Infections: Quinolones are sometimes part of treatment regimens for intra-abdominal infections.
6. Prophylaxis: In certain cases, they are used for prophylaxis against anthrax and certain infections in individuals exposed to contaminated environments.

Adverse Effects:

1. Gastrointestinal Distress: Common side effects include nausea, vomiting, diarrhea, and abdominal pain.
2. Tendon Rupture: Quinolones can increase the risk of tendonitis and tendon rupture, particularly in the Achilles tendon.
3. Photosensitivity: Some individuals may experience increased sensitivity to sunlight and skin rash.
4. Central Nervous System Effects: Quinolones can lead to dizziness, headache, and rarely, more serious neurological symptoms.
5. Cardiovascular Effects: There have been reports of abnormal heart rhythms, including QT interval prolongation.
6. Hepatotoxicity: Elevated liver enzymes and, in rare cases, liver damage may occur.
7. Allergic Reactions: Allergic responses, including skin rashes and anaphylaxis, are possible but not common.
8. Clostridium difficile Infection: As with many antibiotics, quinolones can disrupt the normal gut flora and increase the risk of C. difficile infections.

Nitrofurans

Classification of nitrofurans in table 22 form with their mechanism of action:

Class	Examples	Mechanism of Action
Nitrofurans	Nitrofurantoin, Furazolidone	Nitrofurans work by disrupting bacterial DNA synthesis and damaging the genetic material (DNA) in bacterial cells. They inhibit several enzymes involved in the synthesis of DNA, RNA, and proteins, ultimately leading to bacterial cell death. Nitrofurans are particularly effective against urinary

		tract infections and are active against a broad range of bacteria, including both Gram-positive and Gram-negative organisms.

Metronidazoles

Metronidazoles are effective against a range of anaerobic bacteria and parasites, and they are commonly used to treat conditions like bacterial vaginosis, giardiasis, trichomoniasis, and certain types of infections caused by anaerobic bacteria. Always follow your healthcare provider's guidance when taking antibiotics or antimicrobial medications, including metronidazoles.

Table 23 Classification of Metronidazole, drugs and their mode of action

Class	Examples	Mechanism of Action
Metronidazoles	Metronidazole	Metronidazoles are antimicrobial agents that work by disrupting the DNA and nucleic acid synthesis of microorganisms, including bacteria and parasites. They are particularly effective against anaerobic bacteria and protozoa. Inside the microbial cell, metronidazole undergoes chemical reactions that lead to the formation of toxic compounds. These compounds damage and break the DNA strands, preventing the microorganism from reproducing and ultimately leading to cell death. Metronidazoles are commonly used to treat various infections, including bacterial and parasitic infections.

Glycopeptides

Glycopeptides are critical antibiotics for the treatment of severe bacterial infections caused by gram-positive bacteria, especially when other antibiotics are ineffective. Always follow your healthcare provider's guidance when taking antibiotics or antimicrobial medications, including glycopeptides.

Class	Examples	Mechanism of Action
Glycopeptides	Vancomycin, Teicoplanin	Glycopeptides are antibiotics that primarily target gram-positive bacteria. They work by inhibiting bacterial cell wall synthesis. More specifically, they interfere with the synthesis of peptidoglycan, a critical component of the bacterial cell wall. Glycopeptides bind to the terminal D-Ala-D-Ala residues of the peptidoglycan precursors, preventing them from cross-linking and forming a strong cell wall. This leads to a weakened and structurally compromised bacterial cell wall. As a result, the affected bacteria become more susceptible to osmotic pressure and cell lysis, ultimately leading to their death. Glycopeptides are particularly effective against multidrug-resistant gram-positive bacteria, such as methicillin-resistant Staphylococcus aureus (MRSA). They are used to treat various bacterial infections, including skin and soft tissue infections, endocarditis, and certain respiratory infections.

Oxazolidinones

Oxazolidinones are valuable antibiotics for the treatment of certain bacterial infections. It's important to use them as prescribed by a healthcare provider, and they should only be used to treat infections for which they are specifically indicated. Table 24

Class	Examples	Mechanism of Action
Oxazolidinones	Linezolid	Oxazolidinones, such as Linezolid, are a class of antibiotics that inhibit bacterial protein synthesis by binding to the bacterial 23S ribosomal RNA of the 50S subunit. This binding prevents the formation of the initiation complex, leading to the inhibition of protein synthesis. Oxazolidinones are active against a wide range of gram-positive bacteria, including drug-resistant strains like methicillin-resistant Staphylococcus aureus (MRSA) and vancomycin-resistant enterococci (VRE). They are used to treat various infections, including skin and soft tissue infections, pneumonia, and complicated intra-abdominal infections caused by susceptible bacteria.

AGENTS USED FOR TREATMENT OF FUNGUS INFECTIONS

Fungal infections, often referred to as mycoses, are a diverse group of infections caused by fungi. These infections can affect various parts of the body, including the skin, nails, respiratory tract, and internal organs. Fungi are microorganisms that are distinct from bacteria and viruses, and they can cause a wide range of diseases in humans.

Fungal infections can occur in individuals of all ages and backgrounds. Some fungi are part of the normal human flora, residing on the skin and in various mucosal surfaces without causing harm. However, under certain conditions, such as a weakened immune system or a change in the body's environment, these fungi can become pathogenic and lead to infections.

The clinical presentation and severity of fungal infections can vary significantly. They can range from mild, superficial infections, like athlete's foot or nail fungus, to severe, life-threatening systemic infections affecting vital organs. The choice of treatment depends on the type of fungal infection, its location, and the patient's overall health. Few drugs are available to treat common fungal diseases because most fungi are resistant to common antibacterial drugs. Amphotericin B and the azoles (fluconazole, itraconazole and ketoconazole) act against systemic infections and are particularly harmful to fungi because they interact with ergosterol or prevent its formation. The cell membrane of the fungus contains only ergosterol; Cholesterol makes up the bulk of the sterols in human cells.

Various antifungal drugs are used topically for superficial infections caused by dermatophytes and C. albicans. Nystatin is a polyene antibiotic (similar to amphotericin) that binds to ergosterol and affects the structure of fungal membranes.

Nystatin is used orally to clear gastrointestinal fungi in people with compromised immune systems and is often used topically to treat topical candida infections. Other topical antifungals include thenonazoles tolnaftatum and undecylenic acid, and the azoles miconazole and clotrimazole.

Here's a table 25 listing some common antifungal drugs along with their respective drug classes and mode of action:

Drug Class	Examples of Antifungal Drugs	Mode of Action
Polyenes	Amphotericin B	Binds to ergosterol in fungal cell membrane, causing leakage and cell death
	Nystatin	Binds to ergosterol in fungal cell membrane, causing leakage and cell death
Azoles	Fluconazole	Inhibits fungal cytochrome P450 enzyme, leading to decreased ergosterol synthesis
	Itraconazole	Inhibits fungal cytochrome P450 enzyme, leading to decreased ergosterol synthesis
	Voriconazole	Inhibits fungal cytochrome P450 enzyme, leading to decreased ergosterol synthesis
	Ketoconazole	Inhibits fungal cytochrome P450 enzyme, leading to decreased ergosterol synthesis
Allylamines	Terbinafine	Inhibits squalene epoxidase, a key enzyme in ergosterol synthesis
Echinocandins	Caspofungin	Inhibits the synthesis of β-1,3-D-glucan, an essential component of the fungal cell wall
	Micafungin	Inhibits the synthesis of β-1,3-D-glucan, an essential component of the fungal cell wall
	Anidulafungin	Inhibits the synthesis of β-1,3-D-glucan, an essential component of the fungal cell wall
Pyrimidine Analogues	Flucytosine	Converted to fluorouracil in the fungal cell, inhibiting RNA and protein synthesis
Griseofulvin	Griseofulvin	Interferes with fungal mitosis by disrupting microtubule formation

Morpholines	Amorolfine	Alters fungal cell membrane permeability and function
Thiazoles	Tolnaftate	Disrupts fungal cell membrane integrity and function
Ciclopirox	Ciclopirox	Inhibits fungal cell membrane transport and mitochondrial functions

Nystatin is a polyene antibiotic.

Mechanism of action: The drug is **fungistatic** and **fungicidal.** It binds to sterols, especially ergosterol, which is enriched in the membrane of fungi and yeasts. As a result of this binding, the drug appears to form channels in the membrane which allow small molecules to leak out of the cell.

Pharmacokinetics: Nystatin is not absorbed appreciably from the gastrointestinal tract. It is not absorbed from the skin or mucous membranes. It is not employed parenterally. It is poorly soluble and decomposes rapidly in water.

Therapeutic uses: Nystatin is used to treat *Candida* infections of the skin, mucous membranes, and intestinal tract. Thrush (oral candidiasis) and vaginitis are treated by topical application, whereas intestinal candidiasis is treated by oral administration. Nystatin is supplied as an ointment, oral suspension, oral tablets, drops, and powder.

Adverse effects: Occasional gastrointestinal disturbances occur with oral administration.

Laevorinum is a similar drug which also influences trichomonades.

Amphotericin B is a polyene antibiotic related to Nystatin. Amphotericinum is poorly absorbed from the gastrointestinal tract and is usually ad-ministered intravenously as a colloidal suspension, or in some cases in a lipid formulation. The drug is widely distributed to all tissues except the CNS. Elimination is mainly via slow hepatic metabolism; the half-life is approximately 2 weeks. A small fraction of the drug is excreted in the urine, dosage modification is necessary only in extreme renal disfunction. Amphotericin B is not dialyzable.

Mechanism of action: The mechanism of action is the same for Amphotericin B as for Nystatin. The fungicidal action of Amphotericin B is due to its effects on the permeability and transport properties of fungal membranes. Polyenes are molecules with both hydrophilic and lipophilic characteristics, i.e., they are amphipathic. They bind to ergosterol, a sterol specific to fungal cell membranes, and cause the formation of artificial pores. Resistance can occur via a decreased level of – or a structural change in – membrane ergosterol.

Pharmacokinetics. Amphotericin B is absorbed poorly from the gastrointestinal tract. Intravenous administration results in a plasma half-life of about 24 hours. The drug is excreted very slowly in the urine.

Pharmacologic effects: Amphotericin B is a broad-spectrum antifungal agent. *Histoplasma capsulatum, Cryptococcus neoformans, Coccidioides immitis, Candida* species, *Blastomyces dermatitidis,* and some strains of *Aspergillus* and *Sporotrichum* are sensitive. The concentration of Amphotericin B determines whether it is fungistatic or fungicidal.

Therapeutic uses: Amphotericin B is the most effective drug available for systemic fungal infections. It is frequently used for the treatment of life-threatening fungal infections in patient with impaired defense mechanisms (e.g. patients undergoing immunosuppressive therapy or cancer chemotherapy, and patients with AIDS). Amphotericin B is used in the treatment of the following infections: pulmonary, cutaneous, and disseminated forms of blastomycosis; acute pulmonary coccidioidomycosis; pulmonary histoplasmosis; C. neoformans infections – now the most common life-threatening fungal pathogen associated with AIDS; candidiasis, including disseminated forms. Intrathecal infusion may be helpful in the treatment of fungal meningitis.

Adverse effects: All patients receiving Amphotericin B therapy should be hospitalized, at least during the initiation of therapy. Hypersensitivity reactions can occur, including anaphylaxis. Fever, chills, headache, and gastrointestinal

disturbances are common with intravenous administration. Patients usually develop tolerance to these adverse effects with continuing administration of Amphotericin B. Decreased renal function occurs in over 80% of patients treated with Amphotericin B, necessitating close observation. Normochromic normocytic anemia can occur. Thrombophlebitis can occur.

Griseofulvin is produced by *Penicillium griseofulvum.*

Mechanism of action: Griseofulvin binds to polymerized microtubules, disrupting the mitotic spindle. Griseofulvin interferes with microtubule function in dermatophytes and may also inhibit the synthesis and polymerization of nucleic acids. Sensitive dermatophytes take up the drug by an energy-dependent mechanism, and resistance can occur via decrease in this transport. It is fungistatic.

Pharmacokinetics: Oral absorption of Griseofulvin depends on the physical state of the drug – ultramicrosize formulations, which have finer crystals or particles, are more effectively absorbed—and is aided by high-fat foods. The drug is distributed to the stratum corneum, where it binds to keratin. Biliary excretion is responsible for its elimination. Griseofulvin is absorbed in the upper part of the small intestine following oral administration. Most of the drug is eliminated unchanged in the feces. Griseofulvin has a particular affinity for keratin.

Pharmacologic effects: Griseofulvin is active against dermatophytes, including *Microsporum, Epidermophyton,* and *Trichophyton* species. It is ineffective against yeasts.

Therapeutic uses: Because of its affinity for keratin, Griseofulvin is useful for treating mycotic diseases of the skin, hair, and nails, such as tinea capitis, pedis (athlete's foot), cruris, corporis, and circinata. It is given orally; topical use has little effect.

Adverse effects: Extensive clinical use of Griseofulvin has revealed relatively low toxicity. Possible side effects include headache, neurologic alterations, hepatotoxicity, leukopenia, neutropenia, gastrointestinal distress, and skin reactions, including urticaria and photosensitivity.

Synthetic antifungal drugs

Fluconazole

Mechanism of action: Fluconazole is converted within fungal cells (but not in the host's cells) to 5-fluorouracil, a metabolic antagonist which ultimately leads to inhibition of thymidylate synthetase.

Pharmacokinetics: Fluconazole is well absorbed from the gastrointestinal tract and is distributed widely throughout the body, including the cerebrospinal fluid. It is excreted in the urine, mainly in an unmetabolized form.

Pharmacologic effects: The drug is effective against *C. neoformans.* It is effective against some strains of *Candida,* including some *Candida albicans* strains. However, *C. albicans* can become resistant to fiucytosine during therapy.

Therapeutic uses: Although fiucytosine is not as effective as Amphotericin B, it is less toxic and can be administered orally. It is used for systemic infections caused by *C. albicans* and *C. neoformans (Cryptococcus meningitidis).* It is most often used in combination with Amphotericin B. Recently, the value of this combination has been challenged in patients with AIDS having cryptococcal meningitis because of its toxicity.

Adverse effects have included: fatal bone marrow depression, gastrointestinal upset, skin rash, hepatic disfunction.

Azoles

Classification and pharmacokinetics: The azoles used for systemic mycoses include Ketoconazole, fluconazole, itraconazole, and voriconazole. Oral bioavailability is variable (normal gastric acidity is required). Fluconazole and voriconazole are more reliably absorbed via the oral route than the other azoles. The drugs are distributed to most body tissues, but with the exception of fluconazole, drug levels achieved in the CNS are low. Liver metabolism is responsible for the elimination of Ketoconazole, itraconazole, and voriconazole. Fluconazole is eliminated by the kidneys, largely in unchanged form.

Mechanism of action: The azoles interfere with fungal cell membrane permeability by inhibiting the synthesis of ergosterol. These drugs act at the step of14a-demethylation of lanosterol, which is catalyzed by a cytochrome P450 isozyme. With increasing use of azole antifungals, especially for long-term prophylaxis in immunocompromised and neutropenic patients, resistance is occurring, possibly via changes in the sensitivity of the target enzymes.

Therapeutic uses: Ketoconazole has a narrow antifungal spectrum and is considered to be a backup drug for systemic infections caused by certain blastomyces, coccidioides, and histoplasma. Ketoconazole has been used commonly for chronic mucocutaneous candidiasis and when given orally is also effective against dermatophytes. Fluconazole is a drug of choice in esophageal and oropharyngeal candidiasis and for most infections due to coccidioides. A single oral dose usually eradicates vaginal candidiasis. Fluconazole is now the drug of choice for initial and secondary prophylaxis against cryptococcal meningitis and is an alternative drug of choice (with Amphotericin B) in treatment of active disease due to *Cryptococcus neoformans*. The drug is also equivalent to Amphotericin B in candidemia. Itraconazole is currently the drug of choice for systemic infections due to blastomyces and sporothrix and for subcutaneous chromoblastomycosis. Itraconazole is an alternative agent in the treatment of infections caused by aspergillus, coccidioides, cryptococcus, and histoplasma. In esophageal candidiasis the drug is active against some strains resistant to fluconazole. Itraconazole is also active in dermatophytoses. Voriconazole is a new azole with an even wider spectrum of fungal activity than itraconazole. Its clinical usefulness and toxic potential remain to be established.

Adverse effects: Ketoconazole causes: nausea and vomiting are the most common adverse reactions; hepatotoxicity, hypersensitivity reactions (including urticaria or anaphylaxis), and gynecomastia are less common untoward effects; Ketoconazole transiently blocks testosterone synthesis and the adrenal response to corticotrophin; Ketoconazole blocks several cytochrome P-450-related enzyme steps and, therefore, has the potential to interact with drugs metabolized by the microsomal enzyme system. Fluconazole is less toxic than Amphotericin B or Fluconazole and better tolerated than Ketoconazole. Fluconazole should be discontinued in patients with progressive hepatic disfunction. c. Though it has a lower binding affinity for cytochrome P-450 enzymes than Ketoconazole, it may increase serum concentrations of phenytoin, cyclosporine, and oral hypoglycemic drugs and potentiate the effect of warfarin.

Terbinafine

Mechanism of action: Terbinafine inhibits a fungal enzyme, squalene epoxidase. It causes accumulation of toxic levels of squalene, which can interfere with ergosterol synthesis. Terbinafine is fungicidal.

Therapeutic uses and adverse effects: Like Griseofulvin, Terbinafine accumulates in keratin, but it is much more effective than Griseofulvin in onychomycosis. Adverse effects include gastrointestinal upsets, rash, headache, and taste disturbances. Terbinafine does not inhibit cytochrome P450.

Miconazole and Clotrimazole

These imidazole derivatives are used primarily as topical agents. They inhibit the growth of common dermatophytes and yeasts, including *Trichophyton* species, *Epidermophyton floccosum, C. albicans,* and *Malassezia furfur*. They are used for the treatment of ringworm and other skin infections caused by susceptible organisms, and for vulvovaginal candidiasis. Miconazole is also available for parenteral administration in the treatment of severe systemic fungal infections, such as candidiasis, coccidioidomycosis, and cryptococcosis. However, toxicity and limited efficacy restrict its usefulness.

Sulfonamides

The sulfonamides are derivatives of **sulfanilamide**. Derivatives are made by substitutions in the amide of the sulfonamide group. The Sulfonamides are weakly acidic compounds which have a common chemical nucleus resembling *p*-aminobenzoic acid (PABA). Members of this group differ mainly in their pharmacokinetic properties and clinical uses. Pharmacokinetic features include modest tissue penetration, hepatic metabolism, and excretion of both intact drug and acetylated metabolites in the urine. Solubility may be decreased in acidic urine, resulting in precipitation of the drug or its metabolites. The sulfonamides are classified by pharmacokinetics:

I. Sulfonamides which are resorted,

1. Sulfonamides of short action: Sulfadiazine and aethazolum.
2. Sulfonamides of long action: sulfadimethoxinum and sulfapyridazinum.
3. Drugs with ultralong action: sulfalenum.

II. Drugs which are not absorbed: Pthalazoline, Phthazinum, and Sulginum.

III. Drugs for local action: Sulfacylum-natrium, Aethazolum, and Argosulphanum.

IV. Combination therapy: Biseptol (Co-trimoxazolum).

Mechanism of action: Sulfonamides prevent the incorporation of para-aminobenzoic acid (PABA) into folic acid, which in the reduced form is necessary in purine biosynthesis for the transfer of one-carbon units. Susceptible bacteria are those which need PABA because they are incapable of using folic acid directly. Human cells use exogenous folic acid exclusively, and thus, a lack of PABA does not affect them. They can also act as substrates for this enzyme, resulting in the synthesis of nonunctional forms of folic acid.

Trimethoprim - this drug is structurally similar to folic acid. It is a weak base and is trapped in acidic environments, reaching high concentrations in prostatic and vaginal fluids. It is a selective inhibitor of bacterial dihydrofolate reductase which prevents formation of the active tetrahydroform of folic acid.

Trimethoprim + sulfamethoxazole. Trimethoprim is a highly selective inhibitor of the dihydrofolate reductase of lower organisms. The combination is useful for treating *Pneumocystis carinii* pneumonia, an opportunistic infection seen in patients with AIDS.

When the two drugs are used in combination, antimicrobial synergy results from the **sequential blockade** of foliate synthesis. The drug combination is bactericidal against susceptible organisms.

Pharmacokinetics: Sulfonamides are absorbed within minutes following oral administration. They conjugate with plasma proteins and duration of their action depends on the stability of this connection. They are distributed throughout the body water. They diffuse into cerebrospinal fluid. They are metabolized by acetylation of the para-NH2, which negates the antibacterial activity but not the unwanted effects, sulfadimethoxinum is conjugated with glucuronic acid. Excretion is chiefly via the urine within. The urinary solubility of the various sulfonamides and duration of action varies widely.

A large fraction of trimethoprim is excreted unchanged in the urine. The half-life of this drug is similar to that of sulfamethoxazole (10-12 hours).

Pharmacologic effects: Sulfonamides are effective against many gram-positive bacteria, including group A *Streptococcus pyogenes* and *Streptococcus pneumoniae*.

Many gram-negative bacteria are resistant to sulfonamides, but some, such as *Hemophilus influenzae, Escherichia coli* (the organism most often suspect in acute urinary tract infections), *Shigella, Yersinia enterocolitica,* and *Proteus mirabilis,* often are sensitive. Other susceptible organisms include *Bacillus anthracis, Nocardia, Actinomyces,* and *Chlamydia trachomatis,* the agent responsible for trachoma, lymphogranuloma venereum, and inclusion conjunctivitis.

Therapeutic uses: Sulfonamides are the preferred agents for treatment of: acute uncomplicated infections of breathing system, urinary tract infections; nocardiosis. It is used in otholaryngology. They are effective for treatment of malaria, toxoplasmosis when used in combination with pyrimethaminum, malarial with specific antimalarial drugs. They are used in trachoma and inclusion conjunctivitis as an alternative to tetracycline.

Sulfadiazine is rapidly absorbed and rapidly undergoes urinary excretion. Sulfadiazine is now used less often for urinary tract infections. It is useful for treating diseases of breathing system nocardiosis.

Long acting sulphonamides (sulfapyridazinum, sulfadimethoxinum) are rapidly absorbed, slowly excreted. Period of half-excretion 24-48h. Ultra-long action sulfalenum has period of half excretion less than 48 hours.

Biseptol has wider spectrum of action. The combination was designed to delay development of bacterial resistents. Biseptol is used for treatment of genitourinary, gastromtestinal, respiratory tract infections. **Sodium sulfacetamide** is used in case of infections of the eyes. **Pthalazoline** is unabsorbed in the gastromtestinal tract following oral administration, produces changes only on local gut bacteria flora and finds wide use in presurgical bowel sterilization and in treatment of intraabdominal infections.

Adverse effects: About 75% of untoward effects involve the skin with sensitization often being responsible. Conditions produced include: exfoliative dermatitis; Stevens-Johnson syndrome (fever, malaise, and erythema multiforme). Drug fever can occur and is probably due to sensitization. Blood dyscrasias are rare but can occur. Sulfonamidetherapy is stopped immediately if any of the following hematologic conditions develop to a serious extent: acute hemolytic anemia, which is often, but not solely, due to an erythrocytic deficiency of glucose-6-phosphate dehydrogenase activity and is particularly likely to develop in blacks and children; aplastic anemia; agranulocytosis; thrombocytopenia. Eosinophilia may accompany other manifestations of hypersensitivity. Crystalluria is a condition which was seen with the older sulfonamides but rarely occurs with the newer, more soluble agents such as sulfisoxazole, although some renal damage is still possible. Hepatitis, causing focal or diffuse necrosis of the liver, occurs rarely and may be caused by either direct drug toxicity or sensitization. Kernicterus can occur in the newborn because of displacement of bilirubin from plasma albumin.

Quinolones

There are **chinolons of first generation** – Nitroxoline (NTX), which influence gram-positive, gram-negative microorganisms, fungus (complex with ferum ions, disturb oxidative-reductive process). It is used in urological diseases.

Adverse effects: allergy, dyspepsia.

There are **chinolons of second generation**. This quinolone drug acts against many gram-negative organisms (but not proteus or pseudomonas) by mechanisms which may involve acidification or inhibition of the DNA gyrase. Resistance emerges rapidly. The drug is active orally and is excreted in the urine partly unchanged and partly as the inactive glucuronide. Toxic effects include gastrointestinal irritation, glycosuria, skin rashes, phototoxicity, visual disturbances, and the CNS stimulation. Acidum nalidixicum influences gram-negative microorganisms, disturbs nucleic metabolisms and is used in urinary diseases.

Adverse effects: allergy, dyspepsia, and headache.

There are chinolones of third generation: **ofloxacin, ciprofloxacin, pefloxacin, norfloxacin, fleroxacin, enoxacin, gatifloxacin, levofloxacin, lomefloxacin,** and **sparfloxacin.** All of the drugs have good oral bioavailability (antacids may interfere) and penetrate most body tissues. However, norfloxacin does not achieve adequate plasma levels for use in most systemic infections. Elimination of most fluoroquinolones is through the kidneys via active tubular secretion (which can be blocked by probenecid). Dosage reductions are usually needed in renal disfunction. Moxifloxacinum, sparfloxacin, and trovafloxacinum are eliminated partly by hepatic metabolism and also by biliary excretion. Half-lives of fluoroquinolones are usually in the range of 3-8 hours, but the drugs eliminated by nonrenal routes have half-lives in the 10- to 20-hour range.

Mechanism of action: The fluoroquinolones interfere with bacterial DNA synthesis by inhibiting topoisomerase II (DNA gyrase) and topoisomerase IV. They block the relaxation of supercoiled DNA which is catalyzed by DNA gyrase – a step required for normal transcription and duplication. Inhibition of topoisomerase IV by fluoroquinolones interferes with the separation of replicated chromosomal DNA during cell division. Fluoroquinolones are usually bactericidal against susceptible organisms. The quinolones act on DNA gyrase, an enzyme involved in DNA replication. They are rapidly bactericidal. Resistance to the fluoroquinolones does not develop rapidly as it does with nalidixic acid.

Pharmacokinetics: Ofloxacin, norfloxacin and ciprofloxacin are rapidly absorbed when given orally. Their serum elimination half-life is 3-4 hours. The drugs are metabolized in the liver to some extent. They are excreted in the urine via glomerular filtration and tubular secretion. The drugs are widely distributed throughout the body, but concentrations in the cerebrospinal fluid are low.

Pharmacologic effects: Fluoroquinolones are active against many gram-positive and gram-negative bacteria. Additionally, ciprofloxacin, ofloxacin, lomefloxacin are active against some mycobacteria tuberculosis. They are highly active against gonococci, are active against virtually all urinary tract pathogens. They are highly active against bacteria which cause enteritis and against staphylococci, including strains resistant to methicillinum. But they are somewhat less active against *P. aeruginosa* and many streptococci, and they have poor activity against anaerobes.

Therapeutic uses: Fluoroquinolones are indicated for complicated and uncomplicated urinary tract infections, for serious infectious diarrhea; for infections of bones, joints, skin, and soft tissue; and for lower respiratory tract infections, including those in patients with cystic fibrosis.

Adverse effects: Dyspepsia, headache, skin allergy. Quinolones can cause arthropathy in young animals and, therefore, they are not used in patients under age 17, during pregnancy, or in nursing mothers. Crystalluria has occurred rarely, particularly with alkaline urine. Fluoroquinolones are inhibitors of gamma-aminobutyric acid (GABA) and may cause seizures.

AGENTS USED FOR TREATMENT OF TUBERCULOSIS

The incidence of tuberculosis (TB) has been increasing, particularly in patients with AIDS (Acquired Immunodeficiency Syndrome) due to their weakened immune systems, making them more susceptible to TB infection. To combat TB effectively and prevent the development of drug resistance, a combination of drugs is used for treatment. These drugs are categorized into three groups based on their effectiveness and role in TB treatment:

1. Group A (the most effective): Rifampicinum, Isoniazidum and other derivatives of hydrozyde of isonicotinic acids.

2. Group B (less effective than group A): Streptomycini sulfas, Kanamycinumum, Florymycini sulfas, Cycloserine, Amikacinum, Acthinamidum, Protonamidum, Pyranzinamide, Ethambutolumum, Ofloxacinum, Lomefloxacinum, and Moxifloxacinum.

3. Group C (less effective than group B): Natrii paraaminosalicylas, Thiosemi carbazonum.

The chemotherapy of infections caused by *Mycobacteriurn tuberculosis, M leprae,* and *M avium-intracellulare* is complicated by numerous factors, including limited information about the mechanisms of antimycobacterial drug actions; the development of resistance; the intracellular location of mycobacteria; and the chronic nature of mycobacterial disease, which requires protracted drug treatment and is associated with drug toxicities. Chemotherapy of mycobacterial infections almost always involves the use of drug combinations to delay the emergence of resistance and to enhance antimycobacterial efficacy. The major drugs used in tuberculosis are Isoniazid (INH), Rifampicin, ethambutolum, Pyranzinamide. Actions of these agents on *M tuberculosis* are bactericidal or bacteriostatic depending on drug concentration and strain susceptibility. Suppression of *M avium-intracellulare* in the immunocompromised patient also requires multidrug treatment. The primary drug for leprosy is dapsonum, commonly given with Rifampicin or clofaziminum (or both).

Here's a table 26 listing some of the common agents used for the treatment of tuberculosis (TB):

Drug Class	Examples of Drugs	Mode of Action
First-Line Anti-TB Drugs	Isoniazid (INH)	Inhibits mycolic acid synthesis in bacterial cell wall
	Rifampin (RIF)	Inhibits RNA synthesis in bacterial cells
	Pyrazinamide (PZA)	Not fully understood; disrupts bacterial metabolism
	Ethambutol (EMB)	Inhibits arabinosyl transferase enzyme
	Streptomycin (SM)	Inhibits bacterial protein synthesis
Second-Line Anti-TB Drugs	Amikacin	Inhibits bacterial protein synthesis
	Kanamycin	Inhibits bacterial protein synthesis
	Capreomycin	Inhibits bacterial protein synthesis
	Levofloxacin	Inhibits DNA gyrase and topoisomerase IV
	Moxifloxacin	Inhibits DNA gyrase and topoisomerase IV
	Bedaquiline	Inhibits bacterial ATP synthase
	Delamanid	Not fully understood; may disrupt mycolic acid synthesis
	Linezolid	Inhibits bacterial protein synthesis
	Cycloserine	Disrupts bacterial cell wall synthesis
	Ethionamide	Inhibits mycolic acid synthesis in

| | bacterial cell wall |
| | Para-aminosalicylic acid (PAS) | Not fully understood; may inhibit folic acid synthesis |

Isoniazid is the hydrazide of isonicotinic acid and is a pyridine.

Mechanism of action: Isoniazid probably interferes with cellular metabolism, especially the synthesis of mycolic acid, an important constituent of the mycobacterial cell wall. Isoniazid (INH) is a structural congener of pyridoxine. Its mechanism of action involves inhibition of enzymes required for the synthesis of mycolic acids and mycobacterial cell walls. It can inhibit nucleinic metabolism and competite with vitamins B1, B3, B6. Resistance can emerge rapidly if the drug is used alone.

Pharmacokinetics: The drug is well absorbed from the gastrointestinal tract and diffuses readily into all body tissues and body fluids, including cerebrospinal fluid. The plasma concentration and the metabolism of Isoniazid are affected by whether a given patient is a fast or a slow acetylator of the drug, a genetically determined trait. Isoniazid is excreted mainly in the urine. Slow acetylators have a higher concentration of unchanged or free Isoniazid than fast acetylators. The liver metabolism of Isoniazid is by acetylation and is under genetic control. Patients may be fast or slow inactivators of the drug.

Pharmacologic effects: Isoniazid is effective against most tubercle bacilli. It is not effective against many atypical mycobacteria. To prevent mycobacterial resistance, Isoniazid is used in conjunction with other agents.

Therapeutic uses: Isoniazid is the most widely used agent in the treatment and prophylaxis of tuberculosis.

Adverse effects: Up to 20% of patients taking Isoniazid develop elevated serum aminotransferase levels. Severe hepatic injury occurs more frequently in patients over the age of 35, especially in those who drink alcohol daily. Isoniazid is discontinued if symptoms of hepatitis develop or if the aminotransferase activity increases to more than three times normal. Peripheral and the CNS toxicity occur. This toxicity probably results from an increased excretion of pyridoxine induced by Isoniazid, which produces a pyridoxine deficiency. Peripheral neuritis, urinary retention, insomnia, and psychotic episodes can occur. Concurrent pyridoxine administration with Isoniazid prevents most of these complications. Isoniazid can also exacerbate pyridoxine-deficiency anemia and can produce blood dyscrasias. Hypersensitivity reactions (i.e., fever, various rashes) can occur.

Rifampicin belongs to the group of complex macrocyclic antibiotics.

Mechanism of action: Rifampicin inhibits RNA synthesis in bacteria and chlamydiae by binding to DNA-dependent RNA polymerase. Rifampicin – a derivative of rifamycin – is bactericidal against *M tuberculosis*. The drug inhibits DNA-dependent RNA polymerase (encoded by the *rpo* gene) in *M tuberculosis* and many other microorganisms. Resistance via changes in drug sensitivity of the polymerase emerges rapidly if the drug is used alone.

Pharmacokinetics: When given orally, Rifampicin is well absorbed and is distributed to most body tissues, including the CNS. The drug undergoes enterohepatic cycling and is partially metabolized in the liver. Both free drug and metabolites (which are orange-colored) are eliminated mainly in the feces. Rifampicin is well absorbed from the gastrointestinal tract. It is widely distributed in tissues and is excreted mainly through the liver.

Pharmacologic effects: Most gram-positive and many gram-negative microorganisms are sensitive to Rifampicin. Prolonged administration of the drug as the single therapeutic agent promotes the emergence of highly resistant organisms.

Therapeutic uses: Rifampicin is used in the treatment of: tuberculosis (in combination with other agents, often Isoniazid, Pyranzinamide, or ethambutolum); atypical mycobacterial infections; leprosy. Rifampicin is not used for minor infections because of the emergence of Rifampicin-resistant bacteria.

Adverse effects: Urine, sweat, tears, and contact lenses may take on an orange color because of Rifampicin administration; this effect is harmless. Light-chain proteinuria and impaired antibody response may occur. Rifampicin induces hepatic microsomal enzymes and, therefore, affects the half-life of a number of drugs. For example, a decrease in the effect of some anticoagulants and increased metabolism of methadone occur when these agents are administered concomitantly with Rifampicin. Rashes, gastrointestinal disturbances, and renal damage have been reported. Jaundice and severe hepatic disfunction are occasionally produced.

There are semisinthetic drugs – rifabutinum, etc.

Pyranzinamide is the pyrazine analogue of nicotinamide.

Mechanism of action: The mechanism of action of Pyranzinamide is not known; however, its bacteriostatic action appears to require metabolic conversion via pyrazinamidases (encoded by the *pncA* gene) present in *M tuberculosis* involve inhibition of oxygen dependent mycolic acid synthesis. Resistant mycobacteria lack these enzymes, and resistance develops rapidly if the drug is used alone. There is minimal cross-resistance with other antimycobacterial drugs. Ethionamidum and protionamidum are less effective.

Pharmacokinetics: Pyranzinamide is distributed throughout the body after oral administration. It is excreted mainly by glomerular filtration. Pyranzinamide is well absorbed orally and penetrates most body tissues, including the CNS. The drug is partly metabolized to pyrazinoic acid, and both parent molecule and metabolite are excreted in the urine. The plasma half-life of Pyranzinamide is increased in hepatic or renal failure.

Therapeutic uses: Pyranzinamide is now widely used in multiagent short-term therapy of uncomplicated pulmonary tuberculosis.

Adverse effects: Liver function studies are performed before and during therapy, because liver damage can occur. Hyperuricemia and gout can occur.

Ethambutolum is derivative of ethylenimine.

Mechanism of action connected with blocking nucleonic acids synthesis. Resistance to the drug occurs rapidly when it is used alone.

Pharmacokinetics: Ethambutolum is well absorbed from the gastrointestinal tract. It is widely distributed in the body, including the cerebrospinal fluid. Most of an ingested dose is excreted unchanged in urine and feces. Ethambutolum inhibits arabinosyl transferases (encoded by the *embCAB* operon) involved in the synthesis of arabinogalactan, a component of mycobacterial cell walls. Resistance occurs rapidly via mutations in the *emb* gene if the drug is used alone. The drug is well absorbed orally and distributed to most tissues, including the CNS. A large fraction is eliminated unchanged in the urine. Dose reduction is necessary in renal failure.

Pharmacologic effects and therapeutic use: Ethambutolum inhibits many strains of *M. tuberculosis*. It is used in combination with other agents for the treatment of tuberculosis.

Adverse effects: Visual disturbances, including optic neuritis and red-green color-blindness, can occur but are reversible. Hypersensitivity occurs occasionally, resulting in rash or drug fever.

The use of **streptomycinum** in the treatment of tuberculosis has been declining ever since more effective agents became available. When a three-agent combination is used to treat severe forms of tuberculosis (e.g. disseminated or meningeal), streptomycinum may be one of the drugs used seldom. This aminoglycoside is now used more frequently than hitherto because of the growing prevalence of drug-resistant strains of *M tuberculosis*. Streptomycinum is used principally in drug combinations for the treatment of life-threatening tuberculous disease, including meningitis, miliary dissemination, and severe organ tuberculosis. The pharmacodynamic and pharmacokinetic properties of streptomycinum are similar to those of other aminoglycosides. The second-line antimycobacterial drugs are used in cases which are resistant to first-line agents; they are considered second-line drugs because they are no more effective, and their toxicities are often more serious than those of the major drugs.

Amikacin is indicated for treatment of tuberculosis suspected to be caused by streptomycinum-resistant or multidrug-resistant mycobacterial strains. To avoid emergence of resistance, Amikacin should always be used in combination drug regimens.

Ciprofloxacin and ofloxacin are often active against strains of *M tuberculosis* resistant to first-line agents. The fluoroquinolones should always be used in combination regimens with two or more other active agents.

Sodium aminosalicylate is now rarely used because primary resistance is common. In addition, its toxicity includes gastrointestinal irritation, peptic ulceration, hypersensitivity reactions, and effects on kidney, liver, and thyroid function. Other drugs of limited use because of their toxicity include **capreomycin** (ototoxicity, renal disfunction) and **cycloserine** (peripheral neuropathy CNS disfunction).

PHARMACOVIGILANCE

- The science and activities relating to the detection, assessment, understanding and prevention of adverse effects or any other drug related problem.

Drugs

- *"A chemical substance used in the treatment, cure, prevention or diagnosis of disease or used to otherwise enhance physical or mental well-being"*

Adverse Drug Reaction

- Response to a drug which is noxious and unintended, and which occurs at doses normally used in human for the prophylaxis, diagnosis, or therapy of disease, or for modifications of physiological function

History of adverse effects with drugs is as old as use of drugs / remedies for treatment

- 1780 BC Hammurabi Code: *"If a physician makes a large incision with operating knife and kill him, his hands shall be cut off"*
- In 10th Century, adulteration of drugs was penalised
- In 13th Century, Oath of Apothecaries *"drugs should be of such good quality and of such usefulness that he knows, upon his oath, that it will be good and useful for the confection what the physician is making"*

Adverse effects of drugs were recognised as inseparable part of pharmacotherapy

- 1789: Remedio Morbi: The diseases or ailments which often affect people as a result of administration of remedies for therapeutic purpose.
- Treatment related problems: Essential hazards

- 1800's: Calomel (Mercurous chloride) used for yellow fever. Mercurialism was identified as separate entity
- Sulfanilamide disaster
    - In 1937, elixir of sulfanilamide was prepared in diethylene glycol
    - 107 mortalities were reported
- Re-constitution of FDA
    - FDA was established in 1906
    - In 1938, Food, Drug & Cosmetic Act was signed which required safety testing of drugs before marketing
- Thalidomide Story
    - In 1956, Thalidomide was marketed as sedative initially and later for nausea during pregnancy.
    - First safety concern was neuropathy
    - 1960s saw reporting of phocomelia in Europe, Australia and Canada

> **THALIDOMIDE AND CONGENITAL ABNORMALITIES**
>
> Sir,
> Congenital abnormalities are present in approximately 1.5% of babies. In recent months I have observed that the incidence of multiple severe abnormalities in babies delivered of women who were given the drug thalidomide ('Distaval') during pregnancy, as an antiemetic or as a sedative, to be almost 20%.
>   These abnormalities are present in structures developed from mesenchyme, i.e. the bones and musculature of the gut. Bony development seems to be affected in a very striking manner, resulting in polydactyly, syndactyly, and failure of development of long bones (abnormally short femora and radii).
>   Have any of your readers seen similar abnormalities in babies delivered of women who have taken this drug during pregnancy?
>   Hurstville, New South Wales. WG McBride. .˙. In our issue of Dec 2 we included a statement from the Distillers Company (Biochemicals) Ltd. referring to "reports from two overseas sources possibly associating thalidomide ('Distaval') with harmful effects on the fetus in early pregnancy". Pending further investigation, the company decided to withdraw from the market all its preparations containing thalidomide.
>   —Ed.L.

Kefauver-Harris Amendments

- Introduction of details of efficacy analysis was made mandatory
- Standards were set for granting approvals to drugs

- Systematic collection of reports on all types of adverse drug reactions
- Modified timelines for response from FDA
- Establishment of post-marketing surveillance system
- Establishment of GMP
- Good advertising practices
- Regulated marketing of generics

Evolution of Pharmacovigilance

- 1969 saw reporting of mortalities with digitalis but absence of system of communication between physicians
- Di-ethylstilbestrol (DES) for prevention of miscarriage & incidence of vaginal adenocarcinoma
- 1971 saw establishment of International Drug Monitoring Program
- In 1972 National Pharmacovigilance Centres were established to work in collaboration with WHO
- ICH and CIOMS were established later

Pharmacovigilance in India

- Formal drug safety monitoring system was proposed in 1986
- 12 regional centres
- In 1997, WHO Uppsala Monitoring Centre established National Pharmacovigilance Centre at AIIMS, New Delhi and two other centres at Aligarh & Mumbai
- In 2005, National Pharmacovigilance Program sponsored by WHO was launched with Pharmacovigilance Advisory Committee located at CDSCO, New Delhi and other regional, zonal and peripheral centres

Side-effects/Adverse Effects

- Known
- Unknown
- Expected
- Unexpected

Summarising History of Pharmacovigilance with relevance to India

Year	Event
1747	First reported clinical trials by James Lind, proving the effectiveness of lemon juice in preventing scurvy.
1937	Death of 107 children due to sulfanilamide toxicity.
1950	Apalstic anemia reported due to chloramphenicol
1961	Global disaster due to thalidomide toxicity
1963	16th World Health Assembly recognize to rapid action on ADR's
1968	WHO pilot research project for international drug monitoring
1996	Clinical trials of global standards started in India
1997	India joined WHO Adverse Drug Reaction Monitoring Program
1998	Pharmacovigilance initiated in India
2002	67th National Pharmacovigilance Center established in India.
2004-05	National Pharmacovigilance Program launched in India
2005	Conduct of structured clinical trials in India
2009-10	PVPI initiated

➢ Definitions

Term	Definition
Adverse Event (AE)	Any untoward medical occurrence in a Patient or Clinical Trial Subject administered a medicinal product and which does not necessarily have a causal link with the treatment.
Adverse Reaction (AR) Or Adverse Drug Reaction (ADR)	Any untoward and unintended responses to an investigational medicinal product related to any dose administered.
Unexpected Adverse Reaction (UAR)	n adverse reaction, the nature or severity of which is not consistent with the product information eg Investigator Brochure (IB) or Summary of Product Characteristics

Causal Relationship

According to the WHO, the causal relationship between an adverse event and a suspected drug can be: certain

- probable/likely
- possible
- unlikely

- conditional/unclassified
- unassessable/unclassifiable.

Causal assessment is determined based on temporal relationship, alternative explanations, and (if possible) dechallenge and rechallenge.

To determine the causal relationship (i.e., to assess whether the drug caused the AE/ADR), several medical aspects are evaluated. Elements to assess the causal relationship are e.g. drug's half-life, pathological mechanisms, temporal relationship of event to drug administration, dechallenge and rechallenge, concomitant diseases and/or concomitant use of other medicines, previous experience with the drug, and possible alternative explanations for the event.

Regulatory authority

The legal authority that is responsible for regulating all matters relating to drugs and medicinal products (e.g.: EMA, FDA, MHRA)

The activities of regulatory authorities protect, promote, and maintain the health and safety of the public by ensuring proper standards for the profession of medicine

Key PV Issues

- Adverse drug reactions (**ADR**) harm caused by the use of a drug at normal doses
- Medication errors (**ME**) faulty systems/processes/use
- Poor quality medicines counterfeits/sub-standards

The Pioglitazone Story

- Signals from France & Germany about association between urinary bladder cancer & use of pioglitazone
- US issued a warning in product label
- *"PM & the letter"*
- June 2013, CDSCO bans the manufacture, sale & distribution of pioglitazone July 2013, ban was revoked after lots of deliberations

Aim & Scope

Also, according to WHO, pharmacovigilance has four principal aims, they are, improve patient care and safety in relation to the use of medicines, and all medical and paramedical interventions; improve public health and safety in relation to the use of medicines; contribute to the assessment of benefit, harm, effectiveness and risk of medicines, encouraging their safe, rational and more effective (including cost-effective) use; and promote understanding, education and clinical training in pharmacovigilance and its effective communication to health professionals and the public. Pharmacovigilance plays a critical in every phase of the study, and most importantly, in the post-marketing phase. Once the product enters the market, the intake of an investigational product cannot be controlled by the sponsor. However, it is very important for the sponsor to monitor and assess data on its safety aspects. This can be done by a robust pharmacovigilance strategy that is technology-driven and harmonizes with the medicine and regulatory aspects as well. The basic elements of a **pharmacovigilance strategy** are strong SOPs, accurate case study report capturing, updated safety database, speedy signal detection, expedited reporting to regulatory authorities, and lastly, risk management.

However, any strategy will work only if it complies with regulatory authorities. With tragedies that have taken hundreds of lives, the regulatory authorities have made submission of expedited reports for serious and unexpected adverse events mandatory along with confirmed signals occurring in association with the investigational product. Additionally, a working risk management plan along with qualified professionals who follow all the regulatory guidelines, especially the timelines.

Therefore, with the changing **trends in clinical trials** and changing demographics of the patients taking the medicines, outsourcing pharmacovigilance has been the preferred as they have the expertise to centralize data and hence, early identification of risks; ensuring that the ultimate aim, that is, the safety of human health is fulfilled.

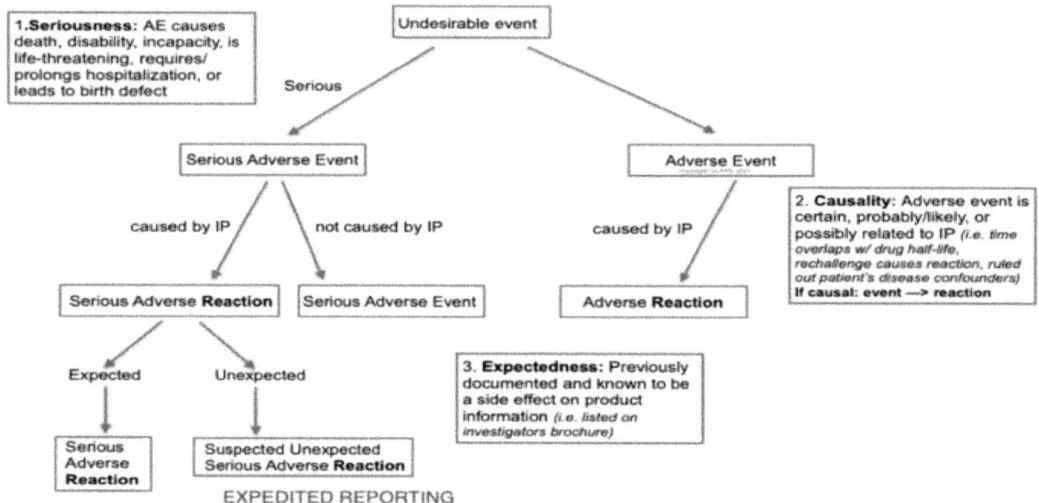

Partners

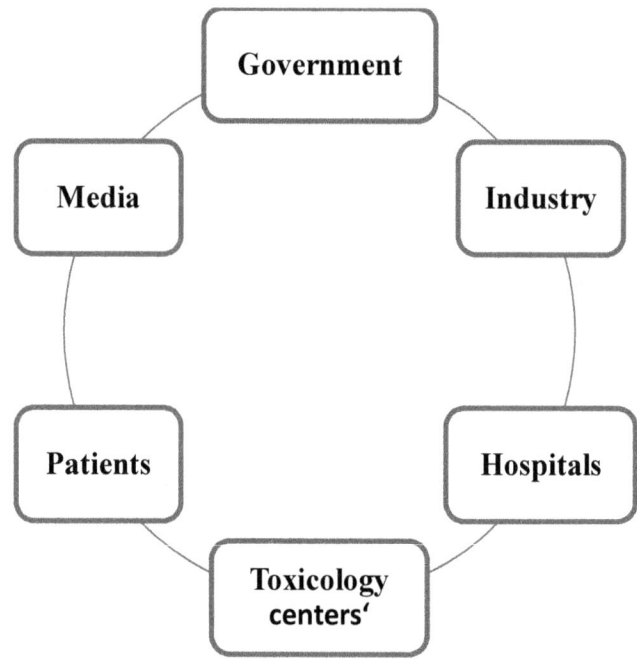

Coding & Software

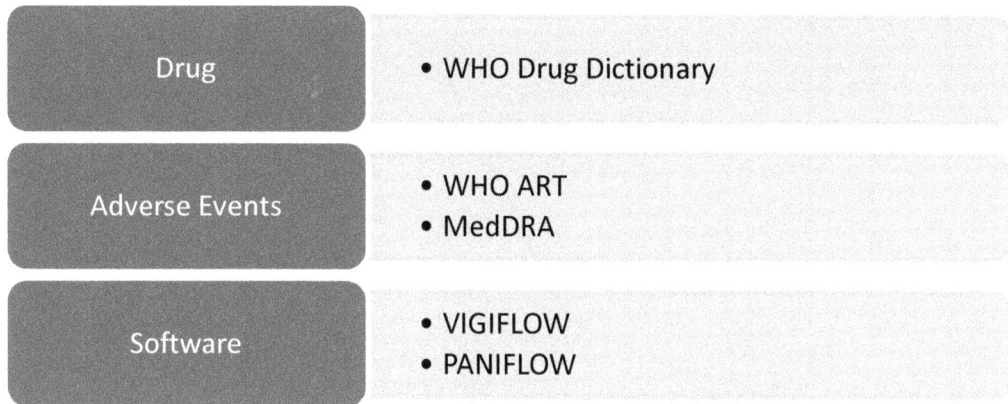

DATA Analysis

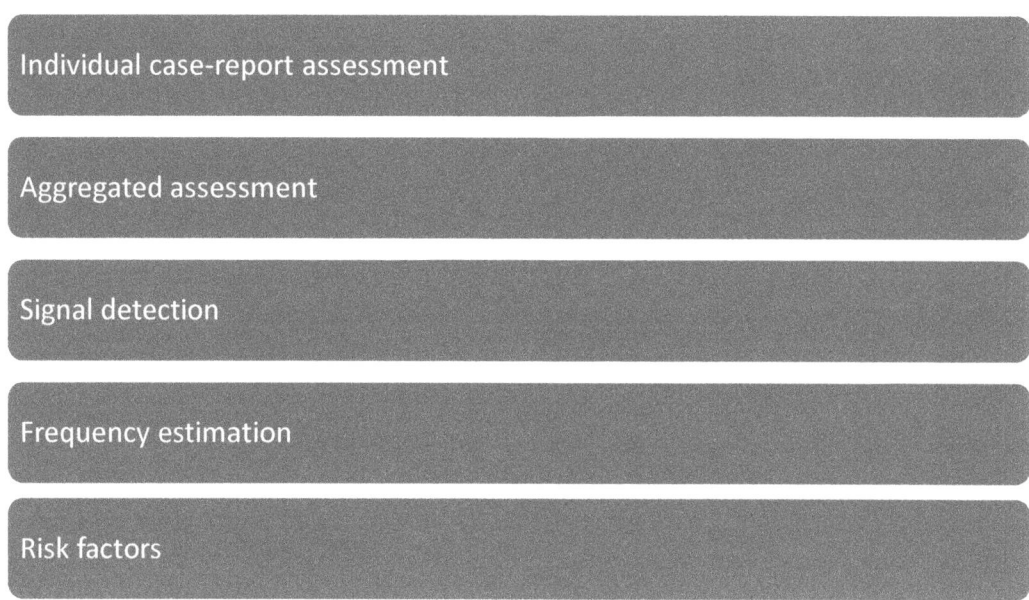

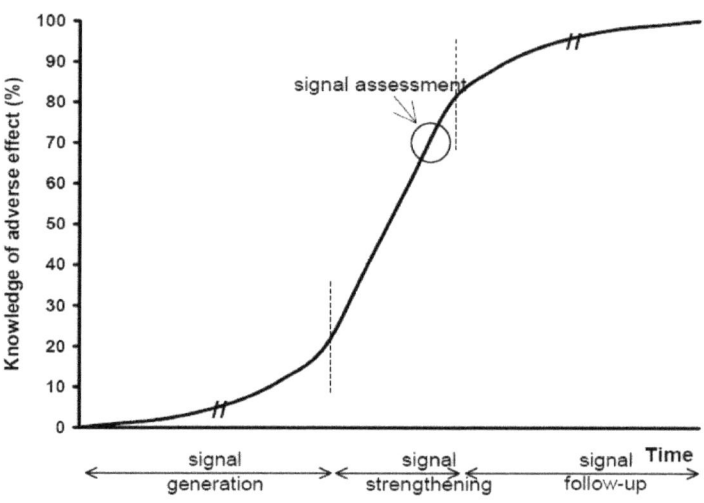

MEDICATION ERROR

"An unintended failure in the treatment process that leads to, or has the potential to harm the patient"

Unintended: To stress on the non-intentional aspect.

Failure: The process has fallen below some attainable benchmark.

Treatment: All treatment not only drugs.

Treatment Process: Starts form manufacturing to consumption of medicines.

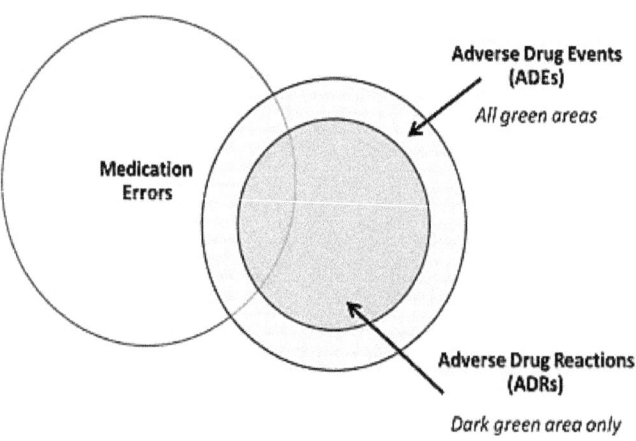

Classification of Medication errors

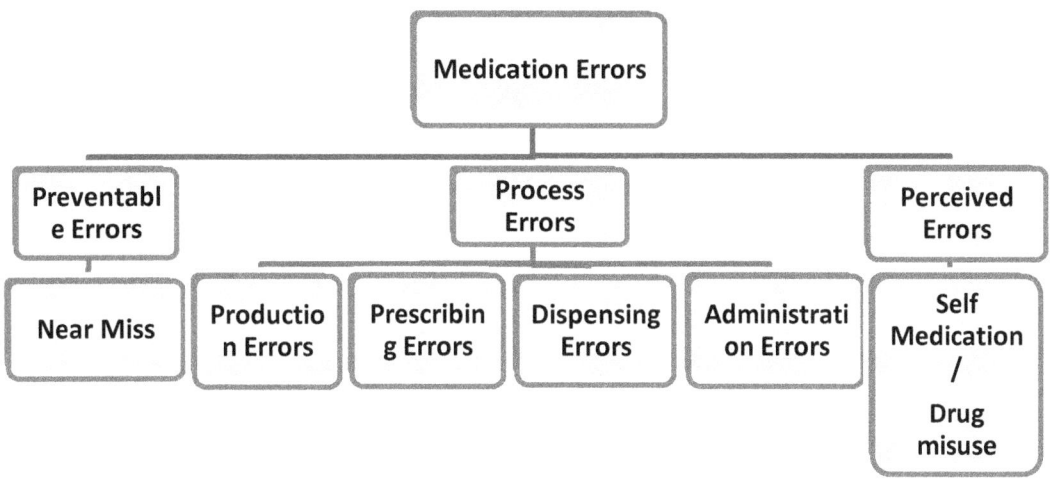

Definitions of terminology used for side effects

Side effect: - Unintended effect occurring at normal dose related to the pharmacological properties.

Adverse Event:- Any untoward medical occurrence in a patient or clinical trial subject administered a medicinal product which does not necessarily have a causal relationship with this treatment. An adverse event can therefore be any unfavourable and unintended sign (e.g. an abnormal laboratory finding), symptom, or disease temporally associated with the use of a medicinal product, whether or not considered related to the medicinal product.

Standard definition of an AE. Important thing to remember here is that it is associated with the use of the product; however, it is not necessarily causally related to the medicinal product. E.g.: a patient took a medicine and fell of a horse accidentally and broke his leg. Breaking his leg would be considered an AE even though it is not related to the medicine.

Serious Adverse Event:- An adverse event which results in death, is life-threatening, requires in-patient hospitalisation or prolongation of existing hospitalisation, results in persistent or significant disability or incapacity, or is a congenital anomaly/birth defect.

In addition to the specific seriousness criteria listed in the definition, medical judgment should be used to assess an AE as serious due to its medical importance. The EudraVigilance Expert Working Group has coordinated the development of an important medical event (IME) terms list based on the Medical Dictionary for Regulatory Activities (MedDRA). This IME list aims to facilitate the seriousness classification of suspected adverse reactions. The seriousness criterion 'Life-threatening' in this context refers to a reaction in which the patient was at risk of death at the time of the reaction; it does not refer to a reaction that hypothetically might have caused death if more severe.

Adverse Drug Reaction:- A response to a medicinal product which is noxious and unintended. Response in this context means that a causal relationship between a medicinal product and an adverse event is at least a reasonable possibility. Adverse reactions may arise from use of the product within or outside the terms of the marketing authorisation or from occupational exposure. Conditions of use outside the marketing authorisation include offlabel use, overdose, misuse, abuse, and medication errors.

Note how ADR differs from AE (above). When we use the word "reaction", we assign at least a reasonable possibility of a causal relationship, whereas the term AE does not imply a causal relationship.

Serious Adverse Reaction:- An adverse reaction which results in death, is life-threatening, requires in-patient hospitalisation or prolongation of existing hospitalisation, results in persistent or significant disability or incapacity, or is a congenital anomaly/birth defect. "Reaction" means that a causal relationship between the medicinal product and the adverse event is at least a reasonable possibility.

Same subtle difference as AE and ADR described above. Any suspected transmission via a medicinal product of an infectious agent is also considered a serious adverse reaction.

Abuse: - Persistent or sporadic, intentional excessive use of medicinal product, which is accompanied by harmful physical or psychological effects. Although being a condition of use outside the marketing authorisation, abuse can lead to ADRs

Medication error: - A medication error is an unintended failure in the drug treatment process that leads to, or has the potential to lead to, harm to the patient. A failure in the drug treatment process does not refer to lack of efficacy of the drug, rather to human or process mediated failures.

This term is related to the way a drug is taken or administered, rather than to the effect it causes. A drug could be wrongly prescribed by a doctor or pharmacist, wrongly dispensed by a nurse or caregiver, or administered incorrectly by a caregiver or patient himself/herself. Although being a condition of use outside the marketing authorisation, medication errors can lead to ADRs. The EMA guidance "Good practice guide on recording, coding, reporting and assessment of medication errors" (EMA/762563/2014, 23 October 2015) points out that medication errors may occur at all stages of the drug treatment process (e.g. prescribing, storage, dispensing, preparation, administration).

Off-label use: - Situations where a medicinal product is intentionally used for a medical purpose not in accordance with the terms of the marketing authorisation.

When drugs are approved by regulators, they get specific approval to use it for a certain indication or population or dose, only. However, sometimes it is noticed that the drug is intentionally prescribed for a medical purpose it is not explicitly indicated for. Examples include the intentional use of a product in situations other than the ones described in the authorised product information, such as:

• Medicine used for disease or medical condition that it is not approved to treat

• Medicine administration through different route or method of administration

• Medicine used with different dose (posology)

• Medicine used in different group of patients (population) Although being a condition of use outside the marketing authorisation, off-label use can lead to ADRs. The element of 'intention' differentiates some of the offlabel uses from the medication error at prescriber level. For example, if the doctor intentionally prescribes/administers a drug by unauthorised route of administration, this would be called off-label use. However, if the doctor unintentionally (i.e. by mistake/error) prescribes/administers a drug by unauthorised route of administration, this would be called a medication error.

Overdose:- Administration of a quantity of a medicinal product given per administration or cumulatively which is above the maximum recommended dose according to the authorised product information. Clinical judgement should always be applied.

As described above there is a maximum permissible dose for every medicinal product. When it is administered above the maximum recommended dose it is considered as an overdose. Although being a condition of use outside the marketing authorisation, overdose can lead to ADRs.

Drug Safety Concepts

Causal relationship: - According to the WHO, the causal relationship between an adverse event and a suspected drug can be:

- Certain
- Probable/likely
- Possible
- Unlikely
- Conditional/unclassified
- Unassessable/unclassifiable.

Causal assessment is determined based on temporal relationship, alternative explanations, and (if possible) dechallenge and rechallenge.

To determine the causal relationship (i.e., to assess whether the drug caused the AE/ADR), several medical aspects are evaluated. Elements to assess the causal relationship are e.g. drug's half-life, pathological mechanisms, temporal relationship of event to drug administration, dechallenge and rechallenge concomitant diseases and/or concomitant use of other medicines, previous experience with the drug, and possible alternative explanations for the event.

Critical terms: - The WHO marked some terms as 'Critical Terms'. These terms either refer to or might be indicative of serious disease states, and warrant special attention, because of their possible association with the risk of serious illness that may lead to more decisive action than reports on other terms. The WHO list of

Critical Terms may serve as a basis for medical judgment of AEs, i.e. to assess whether AEs should be considered serious due to their medical importance.

Important medical event (IME):- The EudraVigilance Expert Working Group has co-ordinated the development of an important medical event (IME) terms list based on the Medical Dictionary for Regulatory Activities (MedDRA). This IME list aims to facilitate the classification of suspected adverse reactions, the analysis of aggregated data and the assessment of ICSRs in the framework of the day-to-day pharmacovigilance activities. The IME list is intended for guidance purposes only and is available on the EMA website to stakeholders who wish to use it for their pharmacovigilance activities. It is regularly updated in line with the latest version of MedDRA.

Efficacy: - The ability of a drug to produce the intended effect as determined by scientific methods, for example in pre-clinical and in clinical research conditions.

Seriousness vs. severity:- The term 'severe' must not be confused with 'serious'. In the English language, 'severe' is used to describe the intensity (severity) of a specific event (mild, moderate or severe); the event itself, however, may be of relatively minor medical significance (such as severe headache). Seriousness (not severity) is based on patient/event outcome or action criteria, and serves as a guide for defining regulatory reporting obligations.

Understanding the difference between seriousness and severity is critical to correctly reporting and evaluating AEs.\

General Pharmacovigilance Terms

CCDS:- Company Core Data Sheet The CCDS is a document that reflects the full company's knowledge and data evaluation for a medicinal product. The safety information contained in the CCDS is referred to as the CCSI (see next definition).

CCSI:- Company Core Safety Information The CCSI is the safety information contained in the CCDS. The CCSI is generally used in all countries where the company markets the medicinal product and is the reference information used to determine listed and unlisted events for the purpose of periodic reporting for marketed products.

DIBD:- Developmental International Birth Date Date of approval of the first authorization for conducting an interventional clinical trial in any country. Determines the start of regulatory requirement. The first data lock point for the DSUR is the first anniversary of the DIBD..

DLP:- Data Lock Point Data lock for data analyses. The DLP represents the cut-off date for data and analyses presented in a document. It is based on the DIBD for the DSURs and on the IBD for PSURs / PBRERs. For RMPs, the DLP can be chosen based e.g. on the cut-off date of the clinical and/or post-marketing data to be included

IB: - Investigator's Brochure The IB is a compilation of the clinical and nonclinical data on the investigational product(s) that are relevant to the study of the product(s) in human subjects. The IB provides the investigators and others involved in the trial with the information to facilitate their understanding of the rationale for, and their compliance with, many key features of the protocol, such as the dose, dose frequency/interval, methods of administration, and safety monitoring procedures. The IB also provides insight to support the clinical management of the study subjects during the course of the clinical trial. For investigational products not yet authorised, the IB serves as the CCDS

Clinical Trail

What Are the Different Phases of a Clinical Trial?

1. Phase I: Doctors give a new treatment to a small number of people to test safety. The researchers find out the best way to give the new treatment, any possible side effects, and safe dosage.

2. Phase II: The research team tries to figure out how well the treatment works for a particular illness.

3. Phase III: The team compares the new treatment with the standard treatment and tries to examine the effects of different dosages and combinations of treatments on different populations (e.g., men, women, young, old, and various ethnic groups).

4. Phase IV: Here, the treatment is tried on average patients who agree to it. The goal is to look for side effects not found in prior phases and to figure out how

well the treatment works over the long term. The FDA allows drugmakers to market the treatment during this phase.

What Are the Advantages of Taking Part in a Clinical Trial?

- You could receive a new treatment before it is widely available to the public.
- You provide researchers with information that helps them come up with better treatments.
- Your treatment costs might decrease because the agency that sponsors the study typically pays for tests and doctor visits related to the trial. It's a good idea to discuss these costs with your medical team before you start.

Could Any Problems Arise From a Clinical Trial Treatment?

Almost all treatments carry some risk. The amount will depend on the type of treatment and on your general health.

In general, scientists don't know as much about how clinical trial treatments affect your body. So there may be more risk of unknown side effects than with already established treatments.

How Does Treatment Differ in a Clinical Trial?

- You may have more exams and tests than usual. These help the research team follow your progress and collect information.
- You may need to stop or change your current medications as well as your diet. Always discuss these changes with your medical team first.
- In some cases you won't know if you get the new medication or something else that looks just like it (double-blind, placebo-control study). This helps the team test how well the drug works.
- Your medical team will ask you to sign documents giving them permission to try the new treatment on you (informed consent).

What Is Informed Consent?

- The doctors and nurses doing the trial will explain the treatment to you, including its possible benefits and risks, and then ask you to sign a release form that gives your consent to take part. This is your "informed consent."

- Keep in mind that your signature does not bind you to the study. You can decide to leave the trial at any time and for any reason.
- In addition, the informed consent process is ongoing. After you agree to a clinical trial, your medical team should continue to update you with any new information about your treatment that might affect your willingness to stay in the trial.

Who Can Take Part in a Clinical Trial?

A trial is typically for a certain condition, and each phase might require a different level of symptoms. If you fit the guidelines for a trial, you may be able to participate. Sometimes you might need certain tests to confirm that you're a good candidate.

Your personal information is confidential and not attached to your name in the study.

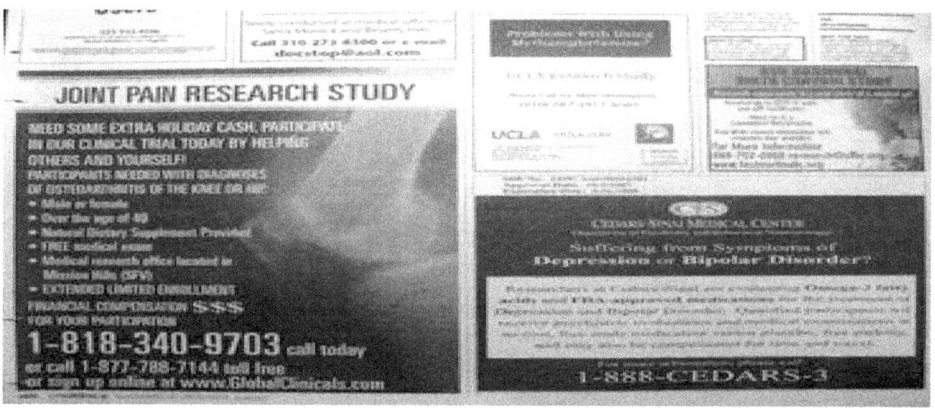

"Newspaper advertisements seeking patients and healthy volunteers to participate in clinical trials"

Phase	Aim	Notes
Phase0	Pharmacodynamics and pharmacokinetics in humans	Phase 0 trials are optional first-in-human trials. Single subtherapeutic doses of the study drug or treatment are given to a small number of subjects (typically 10 to 15) to gather preliminary data on the agent's pharmacodynamics (what the drug does to the body) and pharmacokinetics (what the body does to the drugs). For a test drug, the trial documents the absorption, distribution, metabolization, and clearance (excretion) of the drug, and

		the drug's interactions within the body, to confirm that these appear to be as expected.
Phase I	Screening for safety	Often are first-in-person trials. Testing within a small group of people (typically 20–80) to evaluate safety, determine safe dosage ranges, and identify side effects.
Phase II	Establishing the preliminary efficacy of the drug in a "treatment group", usually against a placebo control group	Phase IIa is specifically designed to assess dosing requirements (how much drug should be given), while a Phase IIb trial is designed to determine efficacy, and studies how well the drug works at the prescribed dose(s), establishing a therapeutic dose range.
Phase III	Final confirmation of safety and efficacy	Testing with large groups of people (typically 1,000–3,000) to confirm its efficacy, evaluate its effectiveness, monitor side effects, compare it to commonly used treatments, and collect information that will allow it to be used safely.
Phase IV	Safety studies during sales	Postmarketing studies delineate risks, benefits, and optimal use. As such, they are ongoing during the drug's lifetime of active medical use.

Appendix-I

APPENDIX-II

List of Banned Drugs by CDSCO

(For details visit www.cdsco.nic.in)

A. Single drug preparations (or combinations of)

1. Amidopyrine
2. Phenacetin
3. Nialamide
4. Methaqualone
5. Methapyriline (and its salts)
6. Practolol
7. Penicillin skin/eye ointment
8. Tetracycline/Oxytetracyline/Demeclocycline liquid oral preparations.
9. Chloral hydrate
10. Dover's powder and Dover's powder tablets I.P.
11. Chloroform exceeding 0.5% w/w or v/v in pharmaceutical preparations.
12. Mepacrine HCl (Quinacrine and its salts) in any dosage form for use for female sterilization or contraception.
13. Fenfluramine
14. Dexfenfluramine
15. Terfenadine

B. Fixed dose combination with any other drug

1. Corticosteroids with any other drug for internal use.
2. Chloramphenicol with any other drug for internal use.
3. Sodium bromide/chloral hydrate with other drugs.
4. Ergot with any drug except preparations containing ergotamine, caffeine, analgesics, antihistamines for treatment of migraine.
5. Anabolic steroids with other drugs.
6. Metoclopramide with other drugs (except with aspirin/paracetamol).

7. Pectin and/or kaolin with any drug which is systematically absorbed from g.i. tract, except for combination of pectin and/or kaolin with drugs not systematically absorbed.
8. Hydroxyquinolines with any other drug except in preparations for external use.
9. Oxyphenbutazone or phenylbutazone with any other drug.
10. Dextropropoxyphene with any other drug except antispasmodics and/or NSAIDs

www.ingramcontent.com/pod-product-compliance
Lightning Source LLC
LaVergne TN
LVHW070521070526
838199LV00072B/6672